Heart Strings

How to Facilitate Heart Health Through the Emotional Anatomy of the Heart

LINDA MARIE

Dedicated, with love to

Grandpa Rob

Who always made time to play

And

Grandma Lily

Who sacrificed her all for family

Other Books By Linda Marie

Archetypes to the Rescue

Your Personal Key Toward Combating Depression

The Art of Sexy Compliments

Using Simple Archetypes to Touch Others

Ruling Energies

Identifying the Powers That Shape Our Lives

The Mysteries of Mistress Energy

Learning How to Break the Allure of Bad Relation-ships and Battle Betrayal

Table of Contents

ACKNOWLEDGMENTS

Sincere appreciation for the patience and intellectual fortitude of Drs. Caroline Myss and C. Norman Shealy, M.D., PhD., my mentors and instructors in the fields of medical intuition, archetype counseling and myriad energy medicine topics through their workshops and at Holos University Graduate Seminary. They are true pioneers of the path less taken.

And to the students in those classes who served as willing guinea pigs and remain close in my heart, especially Vickie.

Health is not valued till sickness comes.

Dr. Thomas Fuller

INTRODUCTION

We live in an age where it is accepted knowledge that emotions can affect physical health. Whether you ascribe to a conventional or alternative healthcare approach, it is generally accepted that there is a mind-body-sprit connection. For decades experiments have been done to achieve results in matter through thought (emotional energy), with overwhelmingly successful results.

You do not have to be a scientist to realize the power a person's thought can have. In 1952, Norman Vincent Peale published his book, "The Power of Positive Thinking." It is a compilation of stories from his life where positive thinking and praying for results lead to positive outcomes.

When I read the book (in the late '80s) I felt that Mrs. Peale was far more positive than Mr. Peale. Now I realize he was writing the book from his own perspective and probably did not want to shade others in clouds of pessimism. Still, credit goes to Mrs. Peale for being a pillar of positive influence. Peale was working on spiritual healing but his work no-doubt opened doors to the myriad connections between emotional and physical well being.

If you are reading *Heart Strings* to get further insight into an ailment that you are experiencing then it would no-doubt help you to get more information about the physical specifics of your area of interest from a medical source. Then, with the understanding of how your body is designed to work and how it is being compromised by the condition you are experiencing, you will be ready to participate with the discussion in

Heart Strings. Once you understand how your thought and emotion affect your heart health you will be able to employ that knowledge as part of your arsenal in your battle to bring your body back to normalcy, or to better cope within the parameters you face. In Chapter Three we will journey into the regions of the heart (and body) that our emotions affect.

Now is a good time to make a clarification: thoughts are perceptions, emotions are feelings. You can have thought without emotion, but it is harder to have emotion (or feeling) without thought. That statement is arguable, and in an argument I would probably land on both sides of the fence (because sometimes thoughts simply can't be put into words and feelings can't be connected to rational thought). For sake of definition in this book let's agree that the words *thought* and *emotion* are interchangeable for we are exploring the relationship of thought-emotion to the heart organ and heart chakra.

It is not a goal of this book to present heart anatomy, but to combine a generalized description of the four chambers of the heart to what I speculate the energetic and emotional connections are in relation to overall health. Be aware that your health concerns may not fall into the groupings that I am forced to make in order to get this information into one book. At times you may feel that your issues reside in a different location. You are the best judge of your mind-body-spirit connection, so feel free to adjust the guidance provided to fit your requirements.

The information you will read will be a diving board for you to use in your own explorations into the unique mind-body-spirit-energy connections that make you unlike any other being on the planet. It may behoove you to get a special journal to record any notes that you feel apply to your situation. More importantly, you may benefit greatly from writing down your feelings as you read. They may lead you to an exploration of personality aspects you have not previously noticed.

LINDA MARIE

HEART STRINGS

*All that is human must
retrograde if it does
not advance.*

Edward Gibbon

CHAPTER ONE

Getting Started

Let's keep this simple. If you are reading
this book, you or a loved one may be dealing
with a heart-related health situation, or you
are an energy worker wishing to add some
tools to your work belt. Since knowledge
cannot serve unless we fully comprehend it,
it is my goal to keep discussion at a basic
level. This book is meant to be the dental
floss in your heart healthcare regime.

As anyone over 30 knows, toothpaste and mouthwash are great, but there comes a time that it will only go so far—deeper cleaning is needed to provide an aging mouth with the care it needs to restore and maintain health. The same thing applies to our physical and emotional health. You have your physician for your physical health; you have me (and other authors) to teach you some approaches to help you with the emotional issues affecting heart health so you can do some deep cleaning and restore your inner harmony.

The number one cause of death in the United States is heart-related disease. It hits our population across the board, which means regardless of age, race, occupation or gender; we are all at risk. It is also as likely for a marathon runner to be at risk as it is for a professional couch potato working on that third chin. It is no wonder that over half of the commercials we see on the television are health related, and that over half of those are heart related.

Every human has death in common but that does not mean we necessarily welcome death, even though we can become the largest obstacles in our fight to maintain a healthy balance. We humans can be our own worst enemies when it comes to caring for ourselves. We continuously get in our own way. It can be easy to see the elephant in the room when standing in someone else's house, but much harder to call it an elephant if looking in the mirror.

Then, once deciding on a productive way forward, we tend to do everything and then look for more to do. Our efforts result in beating ourselves up and burning ourselves out before we get a chance to make any real progress. If we are told "less is more" we simply have to learn not to poke the bear and insist on "more is more." How many of us need two hands to count the number of aerobics videos we own, the number of diets we have tried, the number of exercise programs we have started, or the number of items we have purchased to help optimize health? And, yes, many of those same "have to have" items are now collecting dust in some guilt-locked dark corner of our homes in pristine enough condition to be sold as "new" on Ebay.

There are many things that contribute to heart-related conditions. The medical community advises us to watch our diets by limiting fatty foods and salt intake. We are encouraged to maintain an active lifestyle and to exercise. We are also told to keep our stress levels to a minimum. While this all seems rather simple, our daily lives become so bombarded with "living" that most of the time we do not have two minutes in a day that we can rub together and call our own. The stress of schedules, kids, work, home management, shopping, bill paying, socializing, etc., subtract from the time needed to prepare healthy meals, participate in an exercise program, or to linger in a silent state of meditation.

To all of this confusion and competition for our attention add in the fact that our thoughts and emotions affect our health just as much, if not more than, our physical routines. If we allow ourselves to live lives filled with anger, envy and unforgiveness we risk just as much damage to our heart health as we would if we chose to eat fried foods at every meal.

The physical human body is a complicated system to keep in balance, and so is the human energetic body. We are a mass of electric interchanges; whether it is a nerve firing off pulses or our mind willing our body to react, the energy required to keep each one of us functioning is very real. It is this energy, or electricity, that energy workers can feel, see, or sense, when assessing what is happening within a body.

Do not fall into the illusion though, that only certain people have this kind of talent, because every human is capable of sensing energy. Have you ever had the feeling that someone is watching you only to find out that you were right? Have you ever been drawn to, or repelled by, someone the instant you met? Have you ever had the strong feeling that you should call someone only to have the phone ring and it is that person calling you? Have you ever had the feeling that something was not quite right with your child even though there were no obvious symptoms, only to have him sick a short time later?

The list of how we sense energy is endless. We all do it countless times every day. Some people might name this phenomena *intuition* or *psychic ability*, which would be correct, but we want to be more than intuitive when our heart health is at risk. Working with energy is not the same as merely sensing energy. What do I mean? It is one thing to sense energy but quite another to manipulate or manifest it. It is one thing to see a red aura or feel a cold spot in someone's energy field, and quite another to know what to do with that knowledge. Are you going to learn how to see auras by reading this book? No. There are many other sources and teachers to help you grow into that ability should you wish to learn it. Are you going to learn how to eradicate a cold, red spot? No. Again, there are other teachers for that.

This book is not being created to teach you energy working methodology (even though the suggestions provided are among the techniques used by energy workers). It will, however, teach you how your thoughts help to create dis-ease within your body and where within your heart and body the hurtful energies contributing to heart-related illnesses are stored. With this information will be some energy working suggestions that you can adapt into your health maintenance routines.

You do not have to actively work with energy to reap its benefits. You can get a massage, do yoga, exercise, smile, laugh, pray—the list is long, but be comforted in the knowledge that positive effort reaps positive result. Should you wish to learn how to work with energy there are many modalities from which to choose. A couple of the more hands-on varieties are Reiki and Pranic Healing, both of which can be researched online.

If you are concerned about having "two left feet" when it comes to actually feeling energy you are not unique. There are Reiki masters who do not actually feel the energy they are channeling into a body. In fact, the premise of Reiki work is to treat one's self as a conduit for God energy and to simply focus that energy into another's body at set locations for set amounts of time. Anyone can learn Reiki and successfully use it.

In India the word for energy is *prana*. Grand Master Choa Kok Sui developed and teaches Pranic Healing which helps people learn how to manipulate the energy in our bodies toward our greater good. I have known many people certified in Reiki who studied Pranic Healing and found the latter to open them up to actually feeling energy.

This book is not meant to be a commercial for Reiki or Pranic Healing, but I am often asked how to foster energy reading skills and those are two methods I personally know to work. There are books related to each modality and classes taught in each worldwide.

Energy readers as a rule believe that every human is born with the ability to sense energy fields but that recognition is trained out of existence because it is not acceptable to the societal mainstream. What does that mean? Babies can sense auras, spirits, guardian angels, fluctuations in energy fields that may detect illness, etc. As children grow they are taught what does and does not exist, so if a child says it sees someone/something when an adult cannot, the adult corrects the child leaving it to doubt what it can or cannot clearly see. After being corrected countless times the child starts to believe what it is told to see rather than what it knows to be there. Eventually the child's extrasensory perception is lost.

That does not mean that the sense cannot be revived, but it does take effort and patience. Of course, like any other talent, there will be virtuosos and so-sos. What does that mean? You may spend thousands of hours and even more dollars learning to play the piano, but not everyone who plays the piano is talented enough to be a concert pianist. Does that make your efforts any less useful? If you are willing to be the star of your home parties rather than Carnegie Hall your time will have been well spent.

The same is true with learning and practicing energy work. It is not reasonable to expect perfection when working with energy fields (or anything else for that matter). Whether or not you have extrasensory perception, you can be in-tune with your own body. You can sense when you are "coming down" with an illness or when you just do not feel "right." Depending on how strong the "off" feelings are we seek out our own remedies to bring our bodies back into wellness. Should home remedies not be enough, we know to seek out further assistance.

This book is meant to bring you more weapons for your arsenal against heart-related illness. I will not be able to educate you on every facet of energy work in this book especially since I want to focus on heart-related illness. You are highly encouraged to make your own explorations if terms or modalities are presented that you do not understand. There are many source materials available to you.

So what have we learned? If you have been encouraged to follow a certain health regimen by your doctor, then break it down to the basics and follow that regimen. Do not make it more difficult by adding to it or by trying to do more than the minimum requirements. Why stick to the minimums? Because you may be more apt to stick with the program you have started if you keep it simple. Eventually it will become a habit and your lifestyle will change before you realize it. At that point you may wish to add more to your diet and exercise regimen.

If you know you are at risk then seek professional help, or if it is premature for that much of a step, then work on diet and exercise at your own pace. Hopefully you can also add some energy work into the equation to help work on the roots of your relationship with your heart.

More than anything else, this is a book about relationships. You will be exploring your emotional relationships with yourself and others in an effort to see how your thoughts and feelings are affecting your heart health. You will discover potential thought triggers that may have influenced your heart dis-ease. You will learn about the chambers of the heart where your emotions are processed, which correlate to parts of your body and physical systems. Once you make the connection between how and where your emotions are processed, you will hopefully be able to make your own plan to re-route your thoughts in a more positive direction.

Examples of how to use the information are provided throughout the book. They may not relate to your situation at all, but from the examples you should be able to learn how to tell your own story and then write your own happy ending.

You are about to take a journey—a journey into Self. Before you can hope to understand energy work you must first understand how you relate to, attract, and inhibit, energy within your own being. You must learn to know the difference between energy you generate, energy you give willingly, and energy that is being siphoned from you. You must learn to quit harming yourself through your own thought, and adversely, how to help yourself through thought.

Shakespeare said it best when he wrote, "To thine own self be true." There could be no greater goal in energy work than to know and protect self. Then you will have the luxury of being able to help others.

Homework:

1. Dedicate a notebook and pen (or recording device) to the exploration of your emotional anatomy
2. You may want to make a schedule so you can dedicate specific times for your study
3. When you are doing this energy work ensure you have water and snacks readily available for energy work can be a drain on your system
4. Before being influenced by me, write down anything you feel is pertinent to your current physical, mental, and spiritual health. [Do you exercise? Do you follow a precise diet? Do you have time for meditation or other things a doctor may have recommended to relieve stress? Are there people or situations in your life causing you concern or anxiety? What kind of relationship do you have with: God? Family? Friends? Co-workers? Finances? Leisure time? Hobbies?

Honesty?]

There is no magic trick to doing the homework, and no one will see it. This exercise is to get you on the path of determining your relationship with heart health and emotion.

Mens agitat molem
(the mind moves matter)

Virgil (Aeneid, book 6, line 727) 19 BCE

CHAPTER TWO

The Emotional Energy System

The body is energy. Thoughts are energy. The physical body needs energy (e.g. food), and a system to manage energy, in order to survive. The emotional body needs energy (e.g. happy thoughts), and a system to manage energy, in order to thrive.

The emotional body manages its energy through a system of energy centers, known as chakras. Chakras manage the complex energy exchanges between physical, mental, emotional and spiritual messages the body receives.

Please do not panic over the term "chakra" if it is new to you. You do not have to use that word if it makes you uncomfortable, but if you want to do more research on the topic you will need to use that term. In the meantime, if you want to call your chakras fuse boxes, filing cabinets, energy centers, circuit breakers, etc., you are encouraged to do so.

Readers who have studied chakras will already know that the number of chakras reported to exist in the human body depends on the source you are studying. Do not let that confuse you, and please do not let a number get in the way of using this information. If your modality has chakras not discussed within this book, (e.g. the ajna, or third eye, in Pranic Healing), then simply add them to the way you do your heart-related healing if you feel it is necessary. You, better than anyone else, will know your relationship with chakras (not mentioned here).

Common to all chakra teaching is the fact that each chakra is designated with a portion of the physical body to manage along with certain emotions it is primarily designed to hold and process. However, chakras do not work independently—there are many energetic links between these energy centers (just as there are between the organs of the physical body). For instance, "control" is primarily a Second Chakra (located one-inch below the belly button) responsibility. That is why people who have the need to (over) control things in this life quite often experience colon discomfort which can, through years of concentrated stress, lead to colon cancer. But, when control is perceived through the eyes of fear (e.g. feeling helpless, plagued with anxieties/phobias), it can materialize in the Forth Chakra as a heart or lung condition. If it chooses to remain in the Second Chakra it may appear as diarrhea, spastic colon, etc.

For the sake of simplicity, this book will focus on the Forth Chakra, also known as the Heart Chakra, but because of the intricate connections between chakras, more than one chakra may be involved with a heart-related illness. The Fourth (Heart)

Chakra is located in the area of the chest that houses the heart and lungs and primarily monitors the energy in that area of the body.

It is also important to note here that students of Eastern philosophies and Chinese medicine will have been taught different concepts in regard to Heart Chakra energy. For example, Chinese medicine teaches that grief lives in the lungs. If you get chest colds (bronchitis, pneumonia, asthma, etc.) when you are processing grief, fear, sadness, loneliness, concern…, then you may want to keep an eye on that relationship. For the purposes of this book, we will concentrate on heart issues.

The Heart Chakra also processes the energies of: forgiveness, love, passion (for our dreams), desire (also 2nd), loyalty, determination, steadfastness, altruism, martyrdom, pride, hate, scheming, betrayal (shared with 2nd chakra), longing, envy, jealousy (also 2nd), commitment, fortitude, nobility, fiendishness, anger, grief, depression (also 3rd, 1st), phobias (also in 6th), fear, etc. Greed and lust are primarily handled within the Second (Sex) Chakra, but when elevated to an overwhelming desire the Heart Chakra will also be engaged.

Heart Strings denotes the connection between our emotional and physical beings. That will be done through layman discussion of the heart, as an organ, along with the circulatory system, which thrives only when the heart is working properly. It is important to note here that the circulatory and skeletal systems are the primary responsibility of the First (Root, Base) Chakra. This means that if you are experiencing issues in your vascular system, it is important for you to explore your First and Fourth Chakras for answers.

The First Chakra is where your ancestry lives. Your belief system of how the world operates, and what your place in that operation is, radiates from this center. Your relationship with external family members is reflected here, along with the general values you feel apply to you in this lifetime.

The First Chakra is also where energy workers who feel they must be poor in order to keep pure and maintain their "gifts" get into trouble. They turn their backs on ancestral values, deny self and the energy needed to adequately operate the First Chakra and fail to provide a strong foundation for the succeeding chakras to build upon.

Denying the energy needed to operate, whether that energy is in the form of money or not, is denying the abundance God promises all of His creation. People who are contemplating suicide will also have a huge imbalance between their First Chakra and the rest of the chakra system (the First will feel practically nonexistent).

In the interest of time and space I will be abbreviating the break down of the chakras discussed which may not cover the many nuances of each one. Nor will I discuss technical physiological attributes of the heart or its ailments. There are many books published that discuss chakras as energy centers. There are countless books published that discuss the anatomy of the heart in physical terms, and discuss the physical ramifications of illness resultant to failure of this organ to operate at optimum levels. Your doctor may be able to suggest authors for you to explore for your specific concerns.

It will be helpful if you will approach chakra information as if you are an energy worker looking for clues as to why something is not working well for another person (instead of for yourself). Becoming a third person observer will help you be dispassionate enough to let messages through that you need to hear. Pay close attention to reactions you may have to the energies that each chakra possesses.

Those last two sentences may sound like contradictory advice, but energy workers use the reactions from all of their senses to get "hits" for clients. Keep a log of your feelings so you will be able to investigate them later, on your own. If you know yourself to have a personal relationship with one of the energies (e.g. jealousy), then jot down which chakra can be affected by that energy, and explore the positive and negative situations that emotion creates for you.

Later in the book the chakras will be linked to areas of the heart and related illnesses. Having a start on your relationship with the energies that each chakra stores will provide you with more answers on how to improve your heart dis-ease.

First Chakra

Physically this energy center cares for the circulatory and skeletal systems. There are also ties to neurological systems. This is the chakra that holds your ancestry, so that also means that any hereditary afflictions, genetic disorders (e.g. when joints wear down due to age), and to some extent arthritis (especially if it is similar to that of family members), receive, or are denied, energy from the first chakra.

When the First and Fourth Chakras work together they are generally supporting some kind of vascular issue. This would also include blood clots, circulatory issues surrounding broken bones, and issues concerning cholesterol, plaque or other blockages within veins and arteries. High blood pressure issues would also belong to this chakra alignment, not only because it is a vascular illness, but because stress is often tied to heredity and extended family concerns.

The First (Root, Base) Chakra is the storehouse for all of your family connections. The roots of your perceptions; the foundation of your beliefs; the "reasoning" behind what you value at the deepest levels of your being all reside here. If you ascribe to the concept of pastlife, the lessons learned from your past are stored here for retrieval in this lifetime.

The First Chakra is also known as the Base Chakra and the Root Chakra, it is located at the base of the torso (you sit on it). The First Chakra holds the energies of: tenacity, stamina, materialistic values, societal structure, ancestry, obligation, self-denial, close-mindedness, release, fortitude, meekness, boldness, timidity, fear of failure, fear of acceptance, total acceptance, familial loyalty, relationship to abundance, global relationship to charity and world issues, balance, servitude, enslavement, family influences on how you think, suicidal impulses.

So what does this mean? I will give you one scenario to start with, but there is only a slim probability that it will fit your circumstances. Just know that you can write your own example and fit in pieces relevant to your history.

Blake was born in the southern states of America, raised to be polite, respectful, and exhibit unquestioned loyalty to his family. He is a fifth generation KKK member and dutiful to the society and its mandates. His son, Toby, has a mind of his own and is insisting on going to college at an "unacceptable" school. Fellow Klan members are pressuring Blake to be more forceful with Toby. Blake does not want to lose the loving (yet stressed) relationship he has with Toby, but it is clear that Toby is far too liberal to ever abide by the Klan's, or Blake's, edicts.

In this one instance Blake is tempted to go against the Klan, which is putting a lot of outside pressure on him. Blake wants his son to inherit his legacy, yet he can admire Toby's strength of character in forging his own path. The Klan is concerned that Toby might use his insider knowledge to turn against members in some way, so they view him as a direct threat. Blake is also concerned about Toby and if father and son will spend the rest of their time on earth fighting from different sides of an insurmountable fence.

It does not matter what else happens in the story. This is all we need to know to deduce Blake and Toby both run the risk of developing high blood pressure, peripheral artery disease, risk for stroke, and myriad muscular or skeletal illnesses. It might manifest in something as simple as multiple sprains or tennis elbow, but the longer the rift between father and son is allowed to exist (which is another way to say they are both energetically feeding the rift), the more complicated the physical symptoms each may develop.

What does this mean? Father and son are at an empass. Each can no longer respect the choices the other has made. The more the issue is forced the greater the chasm between them. The father may be able to rise above the differences but that will depend upon the son's compliance—the father is incapable of turning his back on generations of moral heritage, especially when he wants to secure his family line.

The son has broken the mold and in order to remain strong he has had to develop a very thick veneer. One might say he learned to hate (or to love himself more than his external family)—his father and all that his legacy represents. It costs a lot of energy to keep hatred alive—energy that the body needs in order to keep healthy balance. The body can operate for a while with no repercussions, but continual withdrawals of energy needed to run a system (chakra), will result in the compromise of that system.

Hatred lives in the heart chakra (and 2nd, 1st), so it is likely that a system supported by the Fourth Chakra will be involved. Since issues controlled in the First Chakra also complicate this issue, the risks run higher that the heart-related issues will be vascular in nature. We could also say that hatred is Second Chakra energy because oftentimes it is driven from failed sexual liaisons (betrayal). In this situation that is not the case, but if it were we might look for problems in the adrenals, kidneys, colon, large intestine or sex organs.

Second Chakra

The Second Chakra is the energy center responsible for the reproductive organs (to include breasts), bladder, adrenals, kidneys, colon and part of the large intestine. Located about an inch below your belly-button, this is the home of your personal value system. To keep that last statement from confusing you with the values held in the First Chakra, the following is provided: your external family (regardless of the circumstances you were raised under) teaches you about values. That does not mean that you continue to adopt those values as you grow and come to make your own life choices. Your family can pre-dispose you to feel and act in ways acceptable to your clan (First), but eventually you will have to decide if you choose to keep those values (Second). Some experts feel you cannot change core values, but when those values are met head-on with solid reasons for adaptation, sincerity to Self wins. For instance: If you were raised in a family where generations have been connected to organized crime, and your value system was taught to follow that path, it would take strong 2nd Chakra energies to break free and be true to your own moral code of earning money or making an honest living.

How does that example differ from the one presented about the father and son in the First Chakra? It could be argued that it is not different at all. The First and Second chakras overlap in some areas and work in concert in others (as does the entire chakra network). The First example depicted generations of KKK membership. The KKK is an organization that stipulates a very unique way of viewing the world and holds its members to supporting that viewpoint.

The Second Chakra example was similar in that a family connection was involved. We learn our moral codes from our families, but we seem to be born with our core values in tact and many psychologists argue that core values cannot be affected by outside sources (and it is almost impossible for the person in question to alter them).

One of the major core values is how we perceive our personal relationship to money. It would still be possible for someone born into a family of crime to love that family, yet insist on making an honest living. It may involve long distance relationships with family to keep the peace, but it is possible to love the people and not the deeds.

However, there is bound to be friction when second chakra values collide. It is not easy to go against what a family wants for an individual. If the family is an organization formed around a philosophy of crime and an individual within the family wants to make an honest living, the two philosophies can breed distrust among members. Energetically the costs can be great when the second chakra is depleted. In men, the libido is affected when money earning abilities are challenged.

The Second Chakra holds: competition; control; judgement (also held in 4th and 5th); lust; sexual passion; betrayal; personal relationship to money issues; personal values; aspects of martyrdom (that revolve around control); jealousy (which can also be in the 4th); loyalty; vampirism (an aspect of greed and lust); greed; dishonesty, lying; anxiety; worry; creativity; nurturing; personal power; charisma (more of a Third Chakra issue); and addiction.

Third Chakra

Home of the ego and responsible for the liver, stomach, pancreas, gall bladder, transverse colon, diaphragm, appendix, and most of the small intestine; located in the solar plexus (just under your ribcage). The energy center for self-esteem; self-confidence; belief in self; ego; pride; career; dreams; aspirations; vanity; charisma; envy; bragging; self-loathing; insecurity; meekness, boldness; procrastination (also in 6th); responsibility; irresponsibility; drive; laziness; inhibition; shyness (also 5th); justice (can be associated with all chakras); curiosity; intelligence (shared with all, this is more common sense and desire to learn); where your gut feeling resides.

While the First Chakra establishes your inherited

foundation, the Third Chakra establishes your foundation with Self. This is where your identity lives—the innermost you that may not easily be seen or appreciated by the world. That is why the solar plexus comes under attack when others confront you with negative energy.

You may have noticed that when people feel threatened, or are closed off to the energy of others, their arms naturally fold around the abdomen (to protect it from the attack of negative energy). Turning the torso away from the negative energy source is also a way to avoid the full impact of the attack. Doing both (covering the solar plexus and turning your side to the danger) is how to energetically thwart a negativity attack, because such attacks are designed to injure the ego.

Jackie is a very sensitive and caring person with a strong need-to-be-needed. Jackie's motivation in almost every task she performs is to please everyone associated with the outcome. Jackie dresses, performs and spends for what she perceives to be the approval of others. She is in a constant battle with herself to determine what does please others because she is not brave enough to ask—she must rely on compliments and the miserly praise of family and co-workers. Second-guessing every decision from what to wear to who to date is causing Jackie mental and physical distress. She suffers from acid reflux and her sugar levels are in the danger zone. Jackie is at risk for diabetes 2 and stomach ulcers.

Jackie finds it impossible to arm herself against the opinions she imagines others to have of her. She loses personal power to the energy of "compliments." We all run the risk of letting our egos get too tied to the need for compliments, or the reverse energy of criticism. Compliments can drain you of energy if you live your life needing to obtain them from others. There is also the letdown that comes after a compliment is received and it was not quite what was expected. What does that mean? If you spent $200.00 (that was supposed to be used on your car payment) on an outfit to wear to a special event hoping for special recognition and the only comment you received was one unenthusiastic, "nice," you would suffer internal agony.

Compliments are double-edged swords if you need them to feel good. The same goes for criticism if it immobilizes your ability to function. The strongest energetic way to live is in a neutral zone where compliments and criticism are acknowledged but powerless to touch your internal being. Another way to look at this is: what is the person's agenda toward you (your energy) when delivering the compliment (or criticism)? Carefully consider whether or not the other person may have an ulterior motive for complimenting (criticizing) you. That person may be using the compliment (criticism) to get to you in some way, either to endear you or to make you weaker (more dependent on the need for approval). Your best defense is to appreciate what has been said for what it is worth and then to let it go—do not absorb it or dwell on it.

Learn to trust in your own counsel and do things to please yourself. Work hard to remove your ego from the things you produce and participate in. Having pride in yourself is only natural and is actually healthy as long as you do not go overboard and fall to pieces if someone else does not share your opinion. "Live and let live" is an ideal mantra for healing depleted Third Chakra energy. If you desire a more international approach, "Cest la vie" (such is life), would also work.

Fifth Chakra

Located in the throat; responsible for the upper bronchial tubes, thyroid, larynx, vocal cords, trachea, Eustachian tube, mandible, tongue, chin, throat muscles, and lower ear tubes. The energetic home for will, judgement (the spur of the moment comments), choice, self-expression, determination, shyness, insecurity, persuasion, and individual voice. *Speak your own mind* could be the mantra for this chakra, yet so many have trouble finding their voice (whether it is literally in one-on-one encounters, or in public forums through speaking or writing).

Creativity lives in the 2nd chakra, yet many artists use voice as a significant part of their talent package. The 2nd and 5th chakras have a direct connection to each other. That is why so many musicians, singers, actors, politicians, and public figures have problems with sexual issues. People who use voice as a major presentation tool (e.g. politicians, teachers, spokespeople, preachers, journalists) may have challenges containing, or sustaining, libido.

What does this mean? The energy it takes to be creative mingles with the energies of short-sighted judgement and persuasion to make a hybrid "Dr. Jekell and Mr. Hyde" energy punch. You get a supercharged mixture, which puts you on the talent expressway, but you are never quite sure if you will take the good or the evil off-ramp. It is as if your engine is revving too fast for your moral compass to get a true reading.

We see examples of lapses in judgement caused by the combination of Second and Fifth Chakra energies quite often. You just have to pick up a tabloid to do your own research. In fact, the paparazzi (journalistic vampires), are shrouded in Second Chakra energy, which is also the chakra vampires feed on, expressed through Fifth Chakra voice.

Vampires need others to feed on to get sustenance. Journalists are vampires by nature of their jobs. There are also energy vampires that feed off of your energy if you let them. Think about it, you probably know an energy vampire. It is that person that makes you feel exhausted after a few hours of exposure. Some energy vampires have no idea they are draining others, some vampires know exactly what they are doing. The knowledgeable ones go after your money, your time, your personality, and anything else they can get. While they target 2nd Chakra energy, they often use their eloquent speeches (5th Chakra) to lure you in.

Identifying vampires is not as easy as you might think; most of them are very subtle. If you have ever been in a relationship where you did all of the giving and your partner did all of the taking, then you have met a vampire. But try not to judge vampires too harshly, because we all have a relationship with the vampire archetype. In our lifetimes there will be times when we are the suckee and the sucker.

Paula is a confident, successful account executive who has no problem speaking out for the interests of her clients. Paula tends to put everyone else's needs ahead of her own and tries to keep the peace within her extended family. Paula's father is very outspoken and judgmental by nature, which puts Paula and her siblings in a perpetual state of walking on eggshells to keep from becoming targets. Paula has just been diagnosed with high blood pressure, even though it is expected she has had the condition for some time.

Paula is stuck between love and loyalty for her extended family (4th and 1st chakras) and the ability to speak out for herself (5th chakra). While she is able to vent internal stress at work as an advocate for her clients, she has no ability to advocate her own interests. Her family is used to her being the mediator and at times, the peacemaker. No one expects her to be the one they have to contend with because Paula is practically impotent when is comes to making any decisions while with family. No one asks her what she wants to do, what she wants to eat, or where she would prefer going because they all know she will not have a clue. When alone she has no problem making informed decisions, but she is rarely alone since all of her extended family live within five miles of each other.

The high blood pressure took a while to manifest because the body compensated for the withdrawal of energy until it could no longer afford the deficit—then the energy had to come from the energy center most responsible for the drain. In this case Paula is paying the debt from a First Chakra system ran by the Fourth Chakra, but that is only paying for the stress that has built up from the differences between the internal and external pressures within Paula's vascular system.

There is a very high probability that Paula will develop some Fifth Chakra health issue (thyroid, sprained vocal chords, chronic hoarse throat, swallowing disorder, etc.) if she does not learn to find a voice within her own family. Paula's biggest challenge will be to conquer her fear of her father's judgment, or in other words her need for his approval. If she could bring herself to speak up to her father, and consciously make decisions within her extended family, she would find the stress on her system eased and may be able to reverse the high blood pressure. If she fails to overcome her fear of the "judge" she will continue to draw judges into her life and may eventually deplete her Fifth Chakra energy to the point of developing aortic, vertebral or carotid artery disorders.

Sixth Chakra

Also known as the Crown Chakra, located in the center of the top of the head, the Sixth Chakra is the home of the mind, logical thinking, rational thought, and our God connection. It monitors the health of the brain, pituitary, hypothalamus, olfactory, limbic system, hair, eyes, most of the ears, and the head. The medulla oblongata is shared with the 5th chakra. Emotional home for: analytical thinking; mental power; fantasy (shared with 2nd); meditation; phobias; anxiety (shared with 3rd, 2nd, 4th); ideas; unrelenting thoughts; dreams; intelligence (the ability to learn); judgment; will (shared with 5th, 4th, 2nd); sarcasm; meanness; planning; spontaneity; procrastination (shared with 3rd); premeditated activities; humor; wit; scheming; goals; focus; intensity; spirituality (shared with 4th); desire for a God connection; vanity (shared with 3rd); paranormal acclivity; attraction to religion; ceremony.

The Sixth Chakra is home for the majority of our senses—sight, hearing, taste (shared with the 5th), and smell (which is the first and strongest sense we develop). Touch is the fifth sense we possess which is carried by our nervous system and maintained primarily within the first chakra, but shared by all chakras. That leaves us with the question of extrasensory perception, which is what we hope to use when doing energy work. Where does that "live?"

Before we examine internalization of extrasensory information we need to determine the source of that information. Why? Because the "where" to some degree determines your spiritual inclination, which will influence how people answer this question. We also need to agree on what extra-sensory information is. Why? Because we need a common ground to start from and a definition will aid in that start. For our purposes let's agree that extrasensory information is anything we "receive" or "perceive" that is not within the scope of the "normal" use of the other five senses. It would include sound, sight, smell, taste and touch that others cannot sense, but added to that is a "knowing" that others do not have.

There are terms for such "gifts" for you to use should you wish to do more research in developing your own talents: clairvoyance is sight; clairaudiance is hearing; kinetic (or tactile) energy is touch, and clairsentience is knowing. Smell and taste are periphery senses in receiving information usually used to help translate the symbology that is received. [Note: Information received is often in the form of symbols that require interpretation, which fall victim to our own perceptions. That is why energy workers cannot claim to be 100% accurate. What do I mean? If you look at someone's body and see a red spot, what does that mean to you? Simply telling a person you see a red spot provides no use-able information (to either of you). The Universe works with us to provide symbols that we in-turn interpret in order to decipher what we are being shown. What red means to one person may not be what it means to another. These differences can be witnessed by the different colors aura cameras produce and interpret, and in how the books on auras differ. Do not become sidetracked by differences. There are many ways to interpret any kind of information, extrasensory perception is no different. You must learn to accept symbology as a language and create your own unique dialog with the Universe.]

You may also want to call extrasensory information intuition or psychic ability. To people whom use those terms there is a difference, but for our purposes let's agree that the terms are interchangeable. For our level of discussion it does not matter, we need only agree that there is information "out there" that some people can readily tap into and that practically anyone can learn to access. For our purposes, extrasensory information is anything not in the mainstream of human knowledge.

That brings us back to the question of source. From where or whom do we receive this extrasensory information? Depending upon your beliefs it may be from God; guardian angels; the great beyond; a spirit contact (channeling); loved ones who have passed (medium); the cosmic flow (Jung); or it is readily available information that everyone can access (agnostic, atheist, pragmatist, scientist).

Your beliefs are not pertinent to gather information from this book, but they are important for you to explore if you are striving to open yourself to extrasensory perception. Why? If you were raised in a strict religious environment, which teaches that paranormal exploration is sinful, then you have more blocks to overcome than your mere ability to access information. Even if you have left that church behind you, there will still be traces of the old belief system in your core and a probability that your family (1st Chakra) is, or was, rooted to those beliefs. Breaking cords your family still clings to is not usually done by mere will alone, you may have to give it time and effort.

Can you overcome a previous belief in order to claim and explore a new one? Yes, if your desire is strong enough. If you have difficulty opening yourself to the paranormal (or whatever you wish to call it), continue to review your roots. You do not have to accept every idea that is "out there" to access the extrasensory information that you do desire to know. If you find the concept of pastlife (etc.) abhorrent, then so be it. You do not have to believe in pastlife, or any other concept you find offensive, to be intuitive or to work with energy.

Something that will help you open your

mind to exploring extrasensory information is developing the ability to become an observer and not a participant. What do I mean? Learn not to judge or involve your opinion when exploring the information you come across as you open yourself to extrasensory information. If someone does believe in pastlife and you do not, then let it be. If someone says she can see ghosts and you do not believe in that, then let it be. We could go on and on. The only thing that should be important to you is what *you* believe, and your ability to remove yourself from judgment in order to keep your mind open to receiving new information.

How you access information is your own business, and once you start to access it there may be such a flood of it that you cannot tell where it came from or how you received it. The more you open yourself to receipt of extrasensory information the more you receive. The more you receive the less important it becomes to dissect the how, what, why, when, and where of the delivery system.

Why is it important for you to explore your spirituality, learn about chakras, ask yourself questions, keep notebooks, etc., to learn about heart-related illness? There is a direct connection between your physical body and how it operates, and your emotional body and how it operates. We learn about the basic functions of the physical body in our academic education, but unless you seek the information, little to nothing is taught to us about the emotional body. At this point of dealing with your health concern an understanding of emotional anatomy is crucial to your well being.

"You" are not an audience of one sitting in front of me having a personal conversation about your immediate situation. "You" are a generic audience of widely varied personalities and myriad heart health concerns. Everything in this book may not apply to you, pass by that information. It will be there should you choose to read it later. Some things in this book may offend you at a spiritual level. My apologies. All I can ask is that you remain open and take from the book what you can to improve on your situation.

No one is asking you to change your belief system, but you are being asked to explore your thoughts and then to relate them to the state of your physical body. What do I mean? After experiencing a divorce when I was much younger I went through quite an adjustment trying to date again—it seemed so foreign to me and to be honest I did not handle myself very well. I became very disillusioned with men and how they viewed women. I was at that age when I wanted to be seen and appreciated for whom I was and not for what was on the surface. I started telling myself that I needed to meet a man who could love me fat. I said it as a joke not really meaning it, but it became a test a man had to pass before I could let myself become interested in getting to know him.

At that time I was physically fit and very active, but that doubt about the sincerity of men had taken hold and lodged deep in the recesses of my being. Now I am overweight, and still I meet men who seem to be interested in me yet objectify women. I have learned the hard way that people will be who they are and I have choice whether I wish to get closer to them or not. I ruined my figure but it was not without gain—I learned the consequences of thought and how it could affect my body.

Emotional energy is an expression of the self that lives within you. Your spirituality, more than any other way you express or access knowledge, is closer to your emotional energy than is your physical energy. What do I mean? It is easier to understand your emotional energy patterns by analyzing your spirituality than it is to understand your physical body by reading a medical book.

Of course we are exploring an intertwined energy triad—no leg of it can stand on its own for the human body to remain healthy. We need to know what is going on physically to identify bodily trouble spots. The next step is to explore the emotional energies that may have led to deficits that caused the trouble spots. Then that knowledge can be filtered through our spiritual self for help with translating symbology, and resolving energetic problems.

Todd was a swimmer in his youth, loved the sport and was good at it, but late in his high school career he developed chronic swimmer's ear. The pain and drainage were so severe that Todd had to eventually give up the sport. Todd cannot remember the specifics, but it was about that time that Todd's father left and Todd's mother became an alcoholic. Both of Todd's parents became unreliable people that could not be trusted to keep promises.

Todd was abandoned more than once at swimming practice, left to walk home six miles to keep what pride he had left. His grades slipped, not only because of emotional stress but because there was never time to do his homework. Todd had wanted to become an engineer, but when he fell behind in math his chances to get into a good school were crushed. When his parents stopped paying bills, his chances of attending any college were lost.

Todd left home as soon as he turned 18 and aimlessly worked in construction. As his skin cooked while he laid roofing in the summers, and his bones froze while he was framing and putting up sheet-rock in the winters, his heart seethed in hatred of his parents. Todd could not afford health or dental insurance so he ignored any health problems unless they were acute (like when his arm was broken by a falling beam, but the boss on that job covered the expenses).

Todd knew he had something wrong with his wisdom teeth but did not have treatment for the abscesses until he passed-out during a job, in the hot heat of summer, and was hauled away in an ambulance. That time the job did not pay the hospital bills and to add insult to injury he was fired. These types of incidents kept plaguing Todd. In his mid-thirties he was still a struggling construction worker living job-to-job, challenged with sinusitis, migraines, ear infections and dental issues.

This is all we need to know about Todd. Almost 20 years after high school he is still blaming his parents for his failures and bad luck in life. Yes, it was very unfortunate that his family disintegrated while he was young. But, if we believe that Todd chose his parents before he incarnated for the probability of what they would offer him in life, then we also believe that what unfolded was part of the contract Todd requested of God.

Todd still had talent, he simply let his desire dwindle when he started to have to work harder to make his dreams come true. Cursing his parents for all they had robbed him of was easier than taking some adult education courses or attending the local community college until he could improve his grades. Todd was denying his logical brain its chance to expand and that part of him was so starved that it started feeding on other areas as a way to get attention.

Todd had learned to shut down his senses at a young age. He could not bear to hear his parent's fighting, so he quit listening. His deep desire to close off his ears was no-doubt connected to his problems with swimmer's ear. His father's departure probably lessened the tension in the house, but it was replaced by broken promises and intentional lies from both parents. He had seen enough of their neglect and heard enough of their lies to make him want to bite nails. There was so much bile in his heart that he could not love them, and ended up not loving anyone, not even himself.

Todd can explore 1st, 3rd, 4th and 6th chakra energies to find his answers. His pride (3rd) may be keeping him from forgiving (4th) his parents (1st) so he can move on with his life. If he could turn his feelings over to a higher power (6th) and ask for help, it would be a huge step toward forgiveness. Once Todd is free of the hatred he will have room for the joy the Universe is so eager to give him. If he could quit mulling over old thoughts (in his heart and in his head), he would have room for new information his logical mind is craving. He would be able to earn his engineering degree and put his talents to work.

Todd needs to ask himself, "Whom do I want writing my future for me? That angry kid who had his dreams crushed years ago, or the man with all of the experience life has taught?" So far Todd has let that wounded child do all of his thinking and feeling for him. How much more fulfilling would his life become if he could just lay all of that old news aside and allow himself to be filled with new, positive ways of thinking?

At some point we are all asked to leave the past behind and look forward to the future. Even successful people are reminded not to rest on their laurels—we are only as good as our next accomplishment. Forgive and forget (your failures). If Todd can learn to look forward will his health problems disappear? Perhaps not, but it would be interesting to see how his health changed in the next five years.

Seventh Chakra

This may be a controversial chakra for some of you because some books teach there are only six chakras; other books teach there are an infinite number, while some have the number somewhere between six and infinity. You will decide for yourself how many there are, or how many you use. We will use the 7th Chakra here because it does have a connection to heart energy. The 7th Chakra is located about 3 to 6 inches above your head, on the border of your innermost personal aura. Some people feel this chakra is in line with the others, some feel it sits to one side or the other of the head. It does not matter; you will know where yours sits. This chakra continues your God connection. It is actually the chakra you use to communicate with your Guides, etc.; that is why you may hear a voice speaking in your ear. Guides cannot actually enter your body but they get as close to your energy field as possible to help you when you request it (and nudge you when you do not).

The 7th Chakra is your access to the Universal Pipeline of Knowledge, where you gain access to information you want to have and add unique ways of your own to use it. Einstein and Jung both believed this "collective" exists, and theorized that there is no original thought, that everything that could possibly be known already exists and we merely borrow from it. Philosophers would add that we take from this pool of knowledge and fashion it for the contemporary audience (of the time).

The human ego may argue that new ideas

spring from us all of the time, how else would we be any better than a caveman? None of this really matters for our discussion. You need only know that your mind accesses "higher" thought about 3" from the brain. Since there are those of you wondering what we need a brain for then, let's nip those thoughts in the bud. Besides using the brain to regulate all of our physical functions, we use the brain as storage for the knowledge we wish to use on our particular journeys.

We may think we desire to know everything there is to know (at times), but that simply is not true. When we humans do not want to know something, we have a remarkable ability to block it out. We store what we intend to use, knowing that we can access other information when needed. In a way, the cyber network is modeled after the Universal network. The PC hard drive would be our brain, storing what we wish to access frequently (and need to operate efficiently), the Web (7th Chakra) is the conduit to the vast flow of information available for access when we seek answers. There are no emotions linked to this chakra; our desire, curiosity, etc., for what is stored here is shared by all of our internal chakras.

Homework:

1. Go back through the chakra descriptions and write down any of the emotions (by chakra) that cause any kind of response in you, or that you know to be primary to your person
2. If you feel you need to add emotional descriptions to the list in the book, then do so in your notebook so you will have a list that better matches your personality; just ensure you indicate which chakra you are including them into
3. Write down a list of your health problems (if you need any reminders check your medicine cabinet for clues)
4. Take your health problems list and group it into the chakras that primarily care for that part of your body
5. Compare your grouped health problems list to your emotional chakra list to see if you feel your health problems and emotions for each chakra belong where they are (it may be too early for you to know this for sure, so you can merely "*" the ones you have doubts about)
6. Choose one of the chakras, perhaps one that you feel has presented you with the most problems, and write an autobiographical "story" that helps to explain your relationship, and subsequent health issues, with that chakra

LINDA MARIE

We improve ourselves by victories over ourself.
There must be contests, and you must win.

Edward Gibbon

CHAPTER THREE

The Energetic Heart

The heart, as an organ, is rather elongated and sits
in the chest cavity at an angle. The veins and arteries attach to it in a network of loops and interchanges that rival many of our freeways. The heart is also
divided into four chambers, but if you were to try
and draw lines between them, it would be hard to

tell where one begins and the other ends. Of course heart surgeons find this puzzle simple to solve, we lay-people may or may not get all of the pieces back together if the drawn lines actually divided the heart. The heart is a truly complex machine, just as the energies are that the heart chakra manages.

If you are studied in medicine, the energetic explanation of how the heart works may differ with your knowledge of how the physical heart works. Please do not let the simplicity of the energy model keep you from hearing its message, for you, more than many others, are in a position to help people understand this energy.

If you are a medical student, perhaps you should close the book now because you need to learn the actual working of the heart before you confuse yourself with how it appears or works energetically.

The Four Chambers of the Heart and InterChakral Relationships

Imagine you have a very simple diagram of a heart organ in front of you. You are looking at the heart from the back, so the front of the heart is away from you. The right side of the heart in front of you correlates with your right side, the left with your left side. The right side of the heart is the "feeding" side of the organ. Clean, oxygenated blood leaves the right side of the heart through arteries. The left side of the heart is the "receiving" side of the organ. Blood polluted with cell waste is carried to this side of the heart through veins. Each of the chambers of the heart has valves closing it off from other sections of the heart and from the blood vessels (arteries and veins) attached to it.

For our purposes we must exchange the blood that is being carried for energy. The right side of the heart is putting energy that has passed through our heart's filter back into our system. The left side or our heart is collecting and processing the old energy we have already spent. The left side of our heart is breaking down and preparing this energy for filtering and assimilation back into our system (this may sound more like a function of the liver to you, but we are talking about energy and not what the actual organs do).

If the left side of the heart is receiving the used energies of joy, love, passion, forgiveness, etc., the filtering and re-energizing process will be simple and fast. Those energies will be light and easy to carry. If the left side of the heart is receiving the used energies of betrayal, bitterness, vengeance, hatred, fear, etc., it will have a much harder time processing them. Those energies are much more dense—thick and sticky or jagged. That is why beginners in energy work can usually feel the energy of anger before they can feel the energy of joy.

Let's pause here a moment to reinforce a point we have discussed elsewhere. I may have misled you by typifying "good and bad" energies in the example I used. Why? Because it was easier for the point I was trying to make. Emotions, however, are neutral energy—it is how we use them that make them negative or positive, dense or light (and even then those are human perceptions). Love can be just as dense as hate if that love is the smothering, controlling, jealous, martyred type of emotion some people think of as love. Joy can be dense if we are taking joy in another's pain; laughter can be dense if we have used it to laugh at or belittle another person; passion can be dense if we have let our desire for something or someone hurt others, etc.

Betrayal can be light if we have used it to do a good deed for someone; bitterness can be light if we have used it in a good purpose. What do I mean? We see spies on television using betrayal as a smokescreen to thwart the bad guys and help good conquer evil. We read about betrayal in novels because it helps us to tell the good guys from the bad guys. We emulate that behavior in our own lives when we stand up for the underdog. It may take some lying or betrayal to make things work, but when we betray another for the sake of the greater good, we use the light values of that emotion (at least within our own bodies).

We can also betray ourselves into believing things that are not the best for us. In that case the energy being processed is basically neutral because as long as we do not know what is happening we have no repercussions from the use of the energy (one translation of that is: ignorance is bliss). Only you can tell, somewhere deep inside, if the energies you have used are dense, light or neutral.

When dense energies are going through the heart for the first time, the left side will not (usually) have a problem processing them. The left side of the heart is designed to handle the processing function. The energy will be cleansed and the right side will dispense light energy back into the body. But for sake of argument, let's say the dense energy has come back around a few times. Now the energy is clouded when it leaves the right side—it is neither purely light nor dense, but is a mixture of both. When it is processed through the different systems of the body (after leaving the heart), those systems will not really know which of the energies they are receiving. Some may get more light than dense, others more dense than light.

Let's imagine that the Third Chakra received more light energy than dense. That would probably mean that the energy was not to the level of threatening our ego or self-esteem yet, so we would have no reason to plan or plot any type of retaliation, and the organs maintained by the Third Chakra will still be functioning well.

On the other hand, the First Chakra received more dense energy than light. That may mean there is agitation among extended family members building up. Since this has been through our system a few times now we are starting to receive some red flags along our vascular system. Because these dense energies are thicker and more jagged than the light ones, they may be sticking to vascular walls, and they like nothing better than to attract each other, so blockages may be starting to form. We are not in any real trouble yet. Light energy can still be dispatched to wash the stubborn dense energy away, but that option may not always be an option for us.

What does that mean? At this point, some laughter and apologies will defray the dense energies. But, if the issues creating the dense energy continue to escalate, it will take more. At that point prayer and forgiveness may still work. What does that mean? One of the major energetic functions of the heart is to help us with forgiveness. Of course there will be the things we ask forgiveness *for,* but there are also the things we must forgive.

We can store hurts in our body for years; there are lots of places for them to hide. Eventually though, we become imbalanced and there is more hurt than there are places for light energies to travel. This is when there has to be a concerted effort made to change the energies being produced within the body. Light energies will have to be employed.

If the issues causing the dense energies still persist, more drastic measures may need to take place. The person may have to physically move residences or remove self from the presence of the cause of whatever is making the First Chakra unable to produce light energy. If the person does not overcome the issues, further health degeneration may result and the heart and vascular (skeletal) systems will probably be the prime targets.

Now you get to start using the things you learned earlier in the book. If you skipped the chapter on chakras, no worries, you can go back and select information that relates to your situation. An important thing to remember as you start though: energy is like a rolling fog—can you really tell where it starts and stops while standing in the middle of it? Trying to force energy into one certain area would be a lot like trying to push fog into a box. So, if I have told you a certain emotion is processed by a certain chakra, and you feel you have issues surrounding that emotion and health concerns in an area managed by another chakra, then put the two together the way it works best for you.

You have my blessings to interchange information so that it works with you and not against you. However, since we can be our own worst enemies, if you do not feel an improvement after sincerely working at your situation, you may want to go back and see if you missed an emotion that may also be part of the root cause of your dis-ease.

Following is the breakdown of corresponding chakras and the areas of the heart organ that primarily manage them (as it is seen energetically). Remember though that chakra emotion is interchangeable, so this breakdown applies mainly to the health systems managed by the chakras, but they also can overlap.

Left Upper Chamber: 4th, 3rd, (2nd)

Right Upper Chamber: 4th, 5th, (6th)

Left Lower Chamber: 4th, 1st, 2nd,(3rd)

Right Lower Chamber: 4th 1st (3rd)

Okay, so now you have this information. It is possibly the most important information this book has to offer, but how do you use it? First, since heart matters are managed within the Heart Chakra, you can benefit from reviewing the energies of the 4th Chakra, to include the section after this one (on the fifth chamber of the heart). Make notes about your personal relationship/challenges with the energies held in the 4th Chakra.

Next, take the information you have about your medical diagnosis and compare it to the breakdown of the sections of the heart. If you know which section of the heart your dis-ease is in, the better you are to see if the information applies to your situation. If you do compare your medical information to the breakdown provided and determine that the chakra provided in the chamber of the heart housing your challenge does not seem to hold the energy you feel is your primary challenge, then adapt the model to fit your situation.

If you feel you have 5th Chakra issues in the Left Lower Heart Chamber, then go for it, but that would make sense because the 5th and 2nd Chakras do have ties to each other. In fact, many who work with chakras feel the 1st and 6th; 2nd and 5th; 3rd and 4th; have ties to each other. I also feel the 7th Chakra has a relationship with the Fifth Chamber of the Heart (discussed later).

Remember, the 7th Chakra is a pool for the Universal information we tap into. There is a lot of information, depending upon your religious affiliation, about the veil between the earth and Heaven, and how thick that veil is. Most people cannot hope to perceive anything without accessing a guide or learning how to pray. But, with work, people who seek what is beyond the veil can reduce the thickness until there is a mere wisp of fabric between the worlds. The 7th Chakra (13th depending upon the source you use) is the chakra where your energy can co-mingle with Universal energy.

You do not, however, have to concern yourself about anything beyond your health, so focus on the information that pertains to you (you can always go back to explore your spiritual beliefs later).

The Left Upper Heart Chamber

Any part of the heart can be affected by illness, but some quadrants are more likely homes for some occurrences. Transient Ischemic Attacks, and Reversible Ischemic Neurological Deficit are two disorders that frequently occur in the left upper heart chamber. This is also the part of the heart that clots tend to end up at. The 2nd and 3rd Chakras are energetically attached to this area of the heart (but of course any of the chakras may have energetic relationships here).

The left side of the heart is the first place (in the heart) that I would look for evidences of Vampire energy. It may seem to you that the blood leaving the heart (the right side) would be a more prime target, but imagine the blood already being compromised; the lack of blood (energy) is felt in this (upper left) chamber. Of course our archetypal vampires are not actually taking blood from our systems, but they are taking energy, and this is where that energy loss will be felt. This would then leave the right side of the heart with a deficit to recoup when it works to energize the blood going back into the body. So, the right side of the heart is also challenged by vampires, but not as directly.

If you are feeling tired or drained, especially after being with other people, perhaps you should review your relationships and determine if any of those people could be vampires. Once you make that determination you can use that information to help you with your heart health. If you are being attacked by a vampire, remember that it needs others' energy to survive (it is not self-sustaining).

You need to be firm when you tell a vampire, "No." Once it gets the message that whining and begging are not going to get you to change your mind, it will go to another source for what it needs.

71

That does not mean that you always have to avoid your vampire, in many cases the vampire will be a person very dear to you. It simply means that you can plan your excursions around the times that you feel extra strong. Then both of you will part happy. Adopt Van Helsing energy; you know you are going into a vampire environment so you go prepared with the weapons you need to survive.

The vampire typically attacks through the 2nd Chakra, which is secondary to this chamber, but we need to discuss 3rd Chakra issues as well. Review all of the energies maintained in the 3rd Chakra and determine which ones may be contributing to your heart dis-ease. Then, work to contain or control that energy.

Chad had a demanding boss who took credit for work done by his entire staff, and punished staff members if superiors criticized products the division produced. Chad hated the working dynamics but loved the job. There were days he actually cringed when seeing the boss in the parking lot. Chad believes that "right will out" so he waits for the day superiors will fire his boss and promote him to head the division. Chad has worked for the company for over 15 years and within his current division for almost 7; he is at the pinnacle his current position can reach, so upper management is his only way forward. He thinks that at the worst, his boss might be promoted which would open up the division for Chad to take over. He is counting the days until he can throw his promotion party.

Then it happened, the magic day came when the boss was no more. Chad was jumping up and down inside anticipating the call from upstairs that would hoist him up his ladder of success. The day progressed but Chad did not, the phone did not ring. Chad debated on whether or not to make the call himself. He spent a night agonizing over what the superiors were doing; he called everyone in his division to gather information, but nobody was wiser. He invested in a new power suit and decided to impress the upper echelon in person early the next morning.

Chad awoke in a great mood until he realized he overdrew his bank account buying the suit, but he figured that was only a momentary set back. After a restless night, Chad pranced into the executive suite like he owned the place. He was just in time to join a meet-and-greet in the executive lobby. Members of the management staff were being introduced to the new division boss, who was then handed off to Chad for escort downstairs—after Chad was asked to introduce himself because no one upstairs could remember his name. Before lunch Chad collapsed and was taken to the hospital.

If this were your story, where would you begin? Chad's work place is certainly not nurturing, as far as we know, but that could just be Chad's impression of the environment. Does it matter if the actual environment is different from Chad's version? If Chad has delusions of grandeur and is not worthy of a promotion, then yes, it does matter, because his health may not improve until he gets his "status" job and it may be beyond his reach.

We all have our perceptions of events and seldom do they match another's. But, if Chad has worked there 15 years and the executives truly do not know his name, he could be working for vampires—management willing to suck employees dry and offer little to nothing in return. [Note that vampires can also be the friendliest of people while they are stalking their prey].

In this case, let's assume that Chad's perceptions are correct and he has the talent to be in charge of his division. This would mean that he has 2nd and 3rd Chakras engaged in his desire for promotion. He would have been competitive (2nd) for the last 15 years and he would have a lot of his ego (3rd) invested in his advancement strategies. It was not his fault that he worked for a vampire, or that the entire executive suite was one big bat cave.

Could he have done anything to prevent this

outcome? He could have tried to circumvent his boss, but that may not have set well with the vampires upstairs. It is important not to make yourself look good through making others look bad, but in this case the boss was abusing his power. That is the true underlying culprit-energy in this story.

Chad learned to handle the vampire boss as far as his work credit went. Chad was not aware of the vampire superiors; if he had been, he may have known to leave the company before investing so many years. Chad's ego is the true victim here; the blow to his 3rd Chakra was not recoverable. His heart was invested in his promotion so his 4th Chakra literally collapsed when it finally hit him that he was passed over for the position.

Could he have prevented this? Chad's ego is driving that car. Chad sees himself in management; he has attached his dreams (4th) to that achievement. He thought he was investing his time into the grooming of that goal; now it has hit him that he may be too old to start over again (3rd); he fears he will never realize his dreams (4th). The collapse is Chad's knee-jerk reaction to his situation; but we must also consider the shock to his 2nd Chakra: he was counting on the financial gain from the promotion and the reward (medal) from winning the race (beating out the competition).

In reality, companies do take into consideration experience garnered through hard work, and Chad does get points for company loyalty. He may find he is very marketable, but he has wounds to heal before he can have a fresh start. If he tries to seek employment with wounds and hatred in his heart he will only attract another situation like the one he left. His challenge is to rise above vampire energy, forgive the past, and look forward to wonderful new opportunities where he is appreciated for his talents. Can he do it? That is up to him, but at this point he has years of pent-up energy to release before he can move forward.

Chad's situation has been long-term so it probably will manifest in a 4th Chakra ailment (heart or lung disease). If his situation had been short-term we might see indicators of 2nd Chakra problems (sciatica, impotence, colon/intestinal issues). Emotionally Chad might feel aggressive, angry, vengeful, betrayed, drained, and too broken to pick up the pieces (for a short duration).

The Left Lower Heart Chamber

This is the location targeted by most of the heart-attacks people experience. It is also the primary location affected by Congestive Heart Failure. It can also be a location for aneurysms, and is usually the area of the heart compromised by high blood pressure. Renovascular Hypertension that affects the kidneys is also housed here (even though there is a connection with the left upper chamber).

You will note that energetically the lower chamber is connected to the 1st and 2nd Chakras. This tells us that the energies surrounding relationships will play a major role in our exploration. But that is not the only area to concentrate on.

One of the major energies held in the 2nd Chakra is creativity. You may feel you have no connection with this energy if you are not an artist, but you may be mistaken. It is important to stretch, bend, fold, etc., chakral energies in multiple ways before you dismiss them.

What if you wanted children and in the process of trying to procreate you discovered that you could not have a child without the help of a fertility clinic? This is not an issue that would come up in the space of a day or even a month. This is an energetic issue that may take years to build up, and then even more time to resolve. It is immensely stressful on an individual and a couple to go through health issues surrounding the topic of procreation.

It is also an issue that not only affects the couple but the entire external family. As hormones spike out of control so do myriad other emotions as

First and Second Chakra energies are stretched to the limit. This is exactly the kind of stress that can cause dis-ease in the heart.

The energetic stress of wanting to create a child is magnified by the stress of unrequited love aimed toward the nonexistent heir. For the sake of argument let's say the situation is complicated by problems with surrogate mothers, the adoption process, etc. This adds more years to the disruptive energy in the 4th, 2nd, and 1st Chakras, and has probably built up several issues with other people that require forgiveness to release pent-up anger.

If you were trying to resolve a situation like this, what would you do? Perhaps make a list of the people that have aggravated you over the years (concerning your conception situation); or a list of the things you repeatedly think about in relation to your problem. This gives you a place to start. You can review these lists and decide if you have things you need to forgive and set free in order to feel less congested or stressed.

Shelly is a meek, timid person struggling to survive on minimum wage while working as a cook. It is hard, hot labor but she does not feel confident doing anything else. Unfortunately she gets fired from almost every job because she lets the other personnel run all over her and her orders either burn or take too long to prepare. She was married years ago but her husband got tired of yelling at her and beating her so he left. Shelly is still waiting on him to come home and she has kept everything the way he likes it for about ten years now.

Shelly used to be able to augment her income by getting leftovers from the places she worked, but with the onset of diabetes 2 her system cannot really tolerate the food. Her budget cannot afford medication or testing so she has to control her glucose levels through her diet, which is also beyond her budget. Shelly used to think she might be able to become a real chef, but that dream passed her by years ago. She thought she was coping well with her life when out of the blue she had a heart attack.

Shelly's heart was compromised in the lower left chamber. What are the energetic issues she might want to address to bring her heart back into harmony? It would be simple to pin this on 1st or 2nd Chakra issues, right? She no-doubt had a hard and possibly abusive childhood to end up with an overly abusive husband, so there are a lot of forgiveness issues causing her problems, right? Perhaps not, she seemed to be happy in her marriage. Maybe that kind of relationship was all she thought she deserved.

Even if Shelly's childhood was perfect with supportive parents, something happened to make her lose all confidence. Poor self-esteem and lack of ego are the true culprits in Shelly's situation, which is why the 3rd Chakra was weakened first. Shelly would benefit most from a boost of confidence and a scholarship to a cooking school where she could gain the training and backbone she needs to help herself back into health.

We must also consider the diabetes; this is a 3rd Chakra dis-ease energetically associated with issues of responsibility. In Shelly's situation she was taking on too much responsibility and living in fear of having to do everything do someone else's specifications. Feelings of having to be responsible for the "world" can bring that energy into the heart chakra.

The odds of something like this happening for Shelly are slim, but the Universe does work in mysterious ways. She needs to get the notice of some earthbound-angel that believes in her enough to give her a chance. At this point it could be argued that trying to be a chef may be too much stress on Shelly's already timid personality. But, giving her praise and the promise of employment may help raise her level of self-respect enough to help counter the diabetes, which will also go a long way toward helping the heart issues.

You may be wondering why I discuss 3rd Chakra issues here when they are listed as primary issues in the Left Upper Heart Chamber; and why I discussed Vampire energy in the Left Upper Heart Chamber section when the 2nd Chakra is listed as primary in the Left Lower Heart Chamber. Good observations. It was done primarily so you wouldn't feel that energetic vampires cause heart attacks, but with that said a person with an active Vampire archetype (character) may push someone to a state of heart attack in order to take his fortune. And, a person of low self-esteem (3rd) may recognize the Vampire but invite it in because he needs the encouragement.

It is important for you to know that you can manipulate the chart in any way you feel supports your situation. I have provided you with a stepping off place, now you can individualize it for your special situation.

Before we leave this chamber of the heart it is important to address Congestive Heart Failure. Forgiveness is an important energy release for any issue affecting heart health, but it is imperative for people challenged with congestive heart failure. This dis-ease seems to hoard old-used up energy and attempt to feed it with huge amounts of new energy as if it were a baby bird daily eating more than its body weight. Energy healers can literally feel the cloud of energy attached to this dis-ease, but anyone can notice it in the speech of the affected person.

These people live in their history; Archetype Consultants would say that they lead with their Victim archetypes. They have 101 sob stories about how someone wronged them and they aren't shy about sharing the stories with anyone at any time. They will get very worked up about something that happened 30 years ago as if it happened in the last 15 minutes. They may also say that it's all in the past now and that they have forgiven the parties involved, but if that were true why would they still be dwelling on the situation?

If you are cringing in guilt because you told a friend some story about your past yesterday (and still had emotion tied to it), don't be too concerned unless you plucked the story out of thin air (and it had nothing to do with what you and your friend were discussing). If you are concerned, do everything in your power to release the energy behind that situation from your body—forgiving those involved is a good step forward. Remember also that forgiving and forgetting goes further than faking the forgiveness and keeping a string tied to the incident.

The Right Upper Heart Chamber

Arteriosclerosis (thickened blood vessels from high blood pressure) and Atherosclerosis (fatty deposits or plaque in veins), are both vascular conditions. We have discussed vascular conditions belonging to 1st Chakra energy, but here this shows up in a chamber of the heart linked to the 5th Chakra.

The stress behind 1st Chakra-related energetic issues does impact the Left Lower Heart Chamber, but the problem does not stay there. The left side of the heart collects and processes energies; the right side of the heart magnifies and recharges energy for recirculation into the body. When the heart pumps this energy it meets with resistance when it cannot flow freely within the vehicle designed to carry it (the vascular system). That resistance then puts pressure on the delivery system (the chamber of the heart pumping it).

Picture if you will a large balloon trying to release its air through a straw that has been chewed shut in places. In our case the balloon is still being filled so it just gets larger while it is struggling to empty itself. Still sounds like a 1st Chakra issue, but in this case it is not. We have to examine what is causing the pressure on the energy within the heart chamber, and that is 5th Chakra energy.

Review what lives in the 5th Chakra: will,

judgement, choice, speaking your truth, etc. This chamber of the heart is "pushing" its energy into the system, it has to work to make itself heard (or it feels it has to). Some of us are better at expressing Self than others; the rest have to work at it. Choice comes easy to some, etc. We could just as easily say stubbornness, bull-headedness, etc., live in the 5th Chakra, because those energies help us project our will.

When we have problems with making our will known there is just as much pressure put on the heart chamber as when we are aggressively assert-ing our will (or judgement, choice, etc.). Since the 5th Chakra is the literal home of the voice, our voice is involved in helping to relieve some of the pres-sure on our system by releasing the energy of the emotions we are trying to express.

What do I mean? If you are yelling your heart chamber will be depleted of energy until it recharges, which is good for balancing out the ener-gy. If you continually repress our need to yell (ex-press anger), you build up pressure in this quadrant of the heart. If you yell continuously, you effective-ly implode this quadrant of the heart (by not giving it time to reenergize), indicative of people with ex-pressed anger issues and type A personalities hav-ing heart dis-ease manifesting in the vascular parts of the heart (needing bypass surgeries) rather than in the interior of the heart (my intuitive opinion not statistically researched). In a way this is connected to how our singing out-loud (discussed in Chapter Seven) helps to balance our chakras—the combination of breathing in and exhaling loud sounds in a joyful way serves to cleanse our system.

In the Right Upper Heart Chamber the same applies. Our system becomes under pressure from all of the things we feel we are forced to keep inside, and then something happens that breaks the dam and we make the choice to let it all out. The heart and the 5th Chakra both benefit (provided we do not go overboard and cause emotional harm to others).

Darla is in the entertainment field; she is the voice of a popular child cartoon character. As a result Darla tends to revert to her child voice when confronted or forced to make uncomfortable decisions. Darla's friend and agent of many years recently died and she was fraught with grief, but forced to make an immediate replacement because her studio contract was up for negotiation within a week.

Darla did not know where to begin looking for an agent, or how, because her original agent was a friend of the family who was an independent operator. To add to her stress, she was also asked to plan the memorial ceremony. Darla had a lot to handle in one week, and to top it off she had to tape the last three episodes of the cartoon show before summer break (in four days). Darla's body responded by contracting laryngitis, and her chest felt as if her heart were breaking.

This is the chamber of the heart most affected by grief because it is the chamber that has close connection with the lungs and it is the chamber of expression. Our energetic emotions are pooled here to reenergize and flow back into the body. Darla was being torn in multiple directions at once and asked to put 100% effort and attention into each. Short of cloning herself she had few options that allowed her to accomplish everything as well as she would hope.

The pressure built up within her to the point that the 5th Chakra shut down, thereby shutting down Darla's voice box. There was not enough energy available within the 5th Chakra to allow Darla to make all of the choices needed for her friend's service; to interview and hire a new agent; to review and renegotiate a new contract; to read and rehearse scripts; and to record three shows (when normally there would only be one).

Add into the equation that Darla does not want to have to replace her agent; her will is refusing to engage the situation (probably out of loyalty to her friend), making it next to impossible for her to make a choice. She probably doubts her judgement (even though this kind of long-term judgement belongs to the 2nd Chakra) because thinking is causing her grief.

In this situation there is little help within Darla's own system. What she needs is time and release from the pressures crashing in on her. She needs someone to stand up for her and contact her studio to create some kind of work-around (perhaps there is some kind of voice stand-in). Darla probably does not know the first thing about planning a funeral service; she needs to contact a good funeral home and pay for an experienced team to handle some of the details for her (with her inputs).

There are other voice actors on her cartoon show; Darla can ask around and find out who is representing her friends in the business. Yes, she does have to make a speedy career decision at a critical time, but the studio may be able to grant an emergency extension of her current contract to enable her more time to select an agent. It would not be in her best interests to accept a studio agent or to review the contract herself.

When we are the most pressed by time is usually when we need time the most. It is not always possible to obtain an extension, but when it is there is no stigma against accepting that extra time. Another form of time that Darla needs is the time to grieve. She must not let herself confuse her loss of a friend with the loss of a part of her career. If that happens she may lose her ability to create cartoon voices.

Eventually Darla will come to the point where her grief has been allowed to be expressed and the 5th Chakra will be replenished with fresh energy. In the meantime the small choices Darla makes will help her release the pressure valve on her emotions and enable her mind and heart to clear. Restoration of her voice may take a bit more time, but confidence in her ability to choose and judge the situations she is facing will help bring her back into balance.

Why didn't Darla have some form of heart dis-ease? It could have easily been written in (as a clot, stroke, or bypass issue) but not all emotional stress and trauma centered around the heart and 4th Chakra issues are going to result in a massive heart episode. Most of the time it's the building of stress-ful events that result in the creation of heart-related issues; like Darla, you may need to learn that block-ages in other chakras (emotions) can cause pressure on your heart (and other organs).

The Right Lower Heart Chamber

Like the upper chamber, this chamber is responsible for pumping out revitalized chakra energy. The Right Lower Heart Chamber facilitates 1st and 3rd Chakra areas, so in a way it mirrors the function of the upper chamber in that vascular issues are even more emphasized by this chamber. The upper chamber covers vascular health for the top half of the body and the lower chamber for the lower half, making it work harder to manage vascular health in the extremities.

Peripheral Artery Disease (PAD), Gout, Arthritis, (etc.) all depend on this chamber of the heart for ease. This is also the chamber where issues surrounding heartburn are processed. Please read the upper chamber information to learn about the relationships to pressure that these two chambers share. This chamber is perhaps even more sensitive to the fluctuations in pressure to the heart.

Our focus though, is the energies of the 1st and 3rd Chakras. The 1st Chakra houses extended family concerns and the 3rd Chakra deals with issues surrounding Self; this would indicate that the frictions between balancing the two would be of paramount concern within this chamber of the heart. Does that mean that there is a tie between PAD and family squabbles? That would be a logical first place to look, and since the heart contains the energy of forgiveness, it may be an indicator that you have some unresolved issues (to forgive).

Could it be that simple? Well, forgiveness is not a simple energy to master (if anyone truly does), but working toward that end may help ease PAD problems. Forgiveness can be a long-distance effort that one does in solitude, never coming into contact with the source, or originator, of the injury. In some instances that is the only way to accomplish the fete.

In families, however, you are not so readily removed from the source of the injury, even if it is a very distant relative. And, if you are (perhaps by death) there are still the immediate relatives of that person that remind you of your injury.

What do I mean? Kerri is a grown woman and mother who feels well-adjusted, but admittedly has a few problems in her relationships with men, to include her husband. After being diagnosed with PAD she did a lot of soul searching. Kerri realized she still held traces of fear and anger toward her once-favorite uncle who fondled her prepubescent body.

When she thinks of the incident now she does a litany of "what ifs" wondering what would have happened if he had not been interrupted. But he was, and she left the incident in her long-ago past. Or did she? At family reunions she is quick to avoid him along with anyone in his family.

There are six of her 1st cousins that do not share in their father's guilt, yet Kerri finds reasons to maintain distance from them as well. Perhaps they did small energetic crimes against Kerri as young children will, but she has not given them a chance to know her as an adult. Now that her uncle has passed, her aunt is eager to keep a relationship with Kerri, but to her own surprise Kerri cannot seem to move past her need to seek distance from this branch of the family tree.

While this example carries vibrations from the 2nd Chakra, the residual energy is not affecting her ability to maintain sexual relationships. Kerri's current issues evolve around her self-imposed alienation from family. We are not required to have personal relationships with every relative we have, and we will certainly have our favorites among family; but when we go out of our way to avoid family it is an indicator that we have not fully processed negative energy.

Yes, you are right, energy is neither negative nor positive in itself, but as we use energy we attach our own vibrations to it and if it remains in our bodies and festers, eventually causing dis-ease, then let's agree to call those festering pools of energy "negative." As long as Kerri feels the necessity to avoid this part of her inherited family, she will have lingering negative energy lurking in her body that may be contributing to her diagnosis of PAD. [note: this "living in past" energy differs from the energy discussed in relation to congestive heart failure because it is not something living in Kerri's present until she is literally put in front of that branch of the family, which is extremely rare in her situation. If she were to have to face this family on a regular basis, and deal with the feelings she is harboring, chances are her inability to forgive those involved would build until it threatened her with congestive heart failure].

If you have similar ailments but have nothing like this in your past, look to the other energies held in the 1st and 3rd Chakras. Vanity, ego, pride, heredity, societal beliefs, loyalty, etc., may be at the root of your issues to explore.

The Fifth Chamber of the Heart

Now I must truly beg the medical community for indulgence. Energetically, there is a fifth chamber to the heart. It rests near the center, slightly closer to the top, than to the bottom, of the heart. Visually, all of the valves open into this area. So if you are standing in the middle of it, it appears as if you are surrounded by opening and closing heart valves. Remarkably, it is a very quiet and airless place to be—a place where time stops.

This is where the soul lives, at least a part of it. The rest of the soul lives in the limbic system, close to the olfactory, near the center of the brain. There have been many disputes over where the soul lives within us, or if it even does. Few doubt that we have a soul, but having a soul seems to be the indicator that humans are more God-like than the rest of creation.

I believe the soul divides so a part handles matters of the heart and a part takes care of logical decision-making. This division is what can cause us so much frustration when we are trying to make a serious decision. We beat ourselves up trying to decide if we are making a wise or a whimsical choice.

The soul tends to move between its two locations, but at the time of death it leaves the body through the head. Some people have reported hearing a "pop" as the soul leaves. Patients on the brink of demise have been weighed before and after death (for over 100 years) to establish how much the soul weighs, which was determined to be an average of 21 grams (about ¾ oz). German scientists recently weighed over 200 dying people and in every case there was a change of exactly $1/3000^{th}$ of an ounce after death. Perhaps the discrepancy in measurements is due to the improvement in measurement tools and available research. I personally feel the nugget to take away from these findings is that the soul is measureable matter.

Whether you wish to ascribe to any of this is your choice, but you know how it feels to close your eyes in a perfectly dark, completely silent room, and to know exactly who you are. "You" are that essence in your soul, and that quiet place you go is near the center of your heart.

Why is it important to know that this place exists? There is a God connection between our bodies and the Universe, whether we choose to acknowledge it or not (you can explore Astral Projection for more information). When we start to open our minds to the receipt of intuitive information we increase the flow in the channel of that connection. Most of that information will go to the head, but it cannot be accepted as an idea until it processes through the other chakras of the body.

The other chakras only get a yes or no vote; the heart chakra actually makes the decision to consider or reject an idea. What is the difference? The Heart Chakra can ask for more information. The Heart Chakra can send it forward for the head

(Crown Chakra) to consider but still reserve the right to cancel forward action. Basically, no course of action is taken before the heart gives its approval, and the heart gets its advice from the soul.

But if the soul is the soul and simply divided into pieces, why not just let the Crown Chakra handle the decisions? To answer that question we must first explore another "given." The two most powerful energies in the Universe are Love and Fear. We are ultimately judged by whether we make our decisions from a place of love or from a place of fear.

What does that mean? If a woman is married to an abusive alcoholic, does she leave or does she stay? Which decision would be best for her energy? The Universe does not care which path she chooses; there are benefits, trials and potential dangers/blessings to either. The important thing to the Universe is whether she is staying out of fear (that she cannot support herself; that she will not find another partner; that she will suffer more if she leaves); or whether she is staying out of love (that she can help him heal if she stays; that she honors her vows more than her challenges; she is too much in love to leave). Or, if she is leaving out of fear (fear of him; fear of failure; fear of abandonment; fear of becoming an alcoholic); or leaving out of love (loves herself too much to endure anymore punishment; knows she can help them both by leaving because he has to help himself).

If her ultimate choice is made from the energy of Love she can graduate past the tribulations of that challenge. If her ultimate choice is made from the energy of Fear she will face tribulation after tribulation until she can realize Fear keeps her trapped (which is one of the missions of Fear). It isn't because Love is punishing her, it's because Love is a choice—we must consciously reach out to Love (because of our gift of free will). Fear requires no effort, we easily fall into it and sometimes habitually stay in the energy of Fear because it can seem simpler in the moment. But, believe it or not, once you make the decision to choose the energy of Love it becomes the path of least resistance, because you have the power of the Universe on your side to help move your perceived mountains.

The Heart Chakra was created to hold the energy of love, and that energy needs to be protected from outside influences when it is required to make a choice. The soul is there to help the heart know that there are no right or wrong, or good or bad, choices. Choices simply point us in directions, and if we need redirection we will receive it. The Universe tries to help us make decisions with our whole heart. The fifth chamber of the heart is provided as that quiet inner sanctuary that we can all go into to reflect on our choices and commune with our soul (as our soul connects with God).

Energetically, the health of the heart's valves can be affected by our (lack of a) relationship with our soul, and by our hesitation to make decisions with love (or by the majority of our choices being made out of fear). Valve health includes heart murmurs and heartburn. If you are experiencing valve problems, the first place to look is your relationship with the energy of love and with your own soul.

It can be argued that Fear is also held in the Heart Chakra, and this true, but of the two energies (Love and Fear), Love is the strongest. Fear may dominate many of the decisions we make, but that is why Love and the Soul are co-located—to help diminish the control Fear has in our lives.

Homework:

1. Review what you wrote for your health problems and chakral areas of interest
2. Make a list of the heart chambers and their related areas of control that you feel contribute to your own heart dis-ease
3. Compare your lists to the diagnosis obtained from your medical doctor
4. Combine this information into a chart that you can use (e.g. columns for: Diagnosis; Heart Chamber; Chakras Involved; Physical Impact from Chakra; Emotional Energies of Chakra)
5. Use your chart to help you embrace the energies and emotions that you need to bring back into balance

HEART STRINGS

A wise man should consider that health is the greatest of human blessings, and learn how by his own thought to derive benefit from his illnesses.

Hippocrates

CHAPTER FOUR

Your Word Is Your Bond

I used to say, "You're driving me crazy, and that's not a long trip!" Then three people I loved dearly contracted Alzheimer's. That was enough to cure me from saying or thinking that ever again (except for educational purposes). Perhaps the Universe put those people on my path to save me from the same fate—only time will tell.

You can always detect the people who have become familiar with energy work concepts. They are the ones that correct others' speech. For instance, "should" becomes a forbidden word. If you feel you "should" do something that puts unrealistic pressure on you. Relaxing and letting life unfold as it will is considered to be a better alternative. It is also considered more appropriate not to limit yourself with "absolutes." So, the words "always" and "never" are discouraged.

Am I telling you to avoid the same phoopahs? Not necessarily, but there is power in our language. Just as someone else's words can make you feel badly towards self, so can your own inner dialog. There are many ways to interpret that last sentence, but we are not just talking about self-esteem issues.

Take a few minutes to explore what you say (either out loud or to yourself) that might be destructive to your health. You will no-doubt find some of your idioms to seem rather innocent on the surface, so much so that you hear them on television or from others on a regular basis. If you wish to do more research you may want to start in the field of neuro-linguistic programming (NLP).

Let me help you get started: "My feet are killing me." This seems rather innocent, and is even used in a Dr. Scholl's commercial, but it would not seem so light-hearted to a diabetes amputee. "You're stepping on my last nerve!" Humorous unless you have MS, MD, or any other neurological disorder.

Start your list, but before we go much further, would non-body related phrases be just as damaging? Judge for yourself: "I hate her." "I'm just waiting for him to die." "You're an idiot." "What a douche bag."

The list of derogatory statements is endless. The personal repercussions also seem to be. It is said that throwing a pebble into a pond causes an infinite number of ripples. Whether you think the ripples would eventually fade or not is irrelevant. The point is that the pebble still causes disturbance. It may not seem like the person making the example statements is at risk. He is simply expressing himself, right? He is entitled to his own opinion, right? He's just tossing an energetic pebble. But who can say for sure that that small pebble didn't result in a Tsunami?

Of course the man is entitled to his expression. But then he is also running the risk of heart-related illness. Hatred, envy, belittling, trying to disturb another's God connection (or curse another in some way), are all emotions with heart chakra connections. Some of the emotions may manifest in other areas of the body, perhaps the brain or abdomen, but the heart is implicated.

Does that mean if we slip up and say something derogatory toward someone that we are doomed to contract some illness? I would like to say, "No," but I have to insert a warning here. If we deliberately set out to hurl hateful words at someone our spirits will pay a price for it. Those words will stay with us and haunt us, and inevitably come back against us in some way. But the original question was about "slipping up." We have all put a foot in our mouth at some point. It is embarrassing and we usually perform some immediate kind of penitence to restore peace.

What if our negative thoughts are toward some generic audience? What do I mean? I once had a part-time job managing the greeting card aisle for a large drug store chain. While this was only one aisle of the store there were probably over 5,000 different card pockets to oversee. It also seemed to be a popular place for people to visit while waiting on prescriptions to be filled. I took the job as a mental diversion and social outlet and loved being able to help someone find that perfect card to express inner thoughts.

It did not take long for me to notice that the card aisle was susceptible to mass destruction. It does not take many errant children, harried shoppers, or ill inattentive customers to make a royal mess. Then there is the damage to the cards, the stolen envelopes, the misplaced inventory from other parts of the store, and the countless people that wanted me to become their personal shoppers throughout the entire store. When the new of the job wore off I noticed myself welling up with inner anger toward faceless people who intentionally worked to abuse my time and make a mess of my pristine card aisle.

But, being the diplomat that I am I had to defend them by reminding myself that a perfectly orderly card aisle might mean that no one was enjoying the cards, and that would be far worse than having to straighten them. My Diplomat was not always heard above the ranting Scribe who needed everything to be in place and for people to respect the cards. The inner dialog became quite graphic at times and that made me wonder why I kept the job. It certainly was not for the 4 to 15 hours of work at minimum wage that I might earn in that week.

It became clear to me that I had to keep the job until I could perform it with joy in my heart regardless of the state of the aisle or the demands from customers. I kept score and if I had one inner thought that was belittling I could not count that day as one I lived in harmony. It was my goal to have three harmonic days in a row (at work) before I could quit the job. Let's just say it took over a year before I succeeded. It was much easier to learn to gather my energy and put myself in "now" space (a fete some energy workers never learn), than it was for me to learn not to throw harpoons at nameless others for the condition of my card aisle.

Truth comes to us in many ways. In fact, some ways to distinguish Truth from mere speculation is that Truth stands the test of time and crosses the spectrum of belief systems. Some Truth travels to us in sayings that make it easier to absorb, define and teach. Some of this truth lives in what we warmly call "Old Wives' Tales." Other truth survives time in cliches we use, or single words we use to encapsulate larger, broader feelings. Some of these words start as names that grow to become symbolic icons.

When was the last time you asked someone for a Kleenex (when that is a brand name for a tissue)? Or, asked for a Post-it when you meant sticky pad? Or, told someone he was "cruising for a bruising" when you were upset? Sometimes brand names become a part of our daily vocabulary, which is wonderful for that particular marketing program. Other times sayings become part of our speech.

For instance, "A penny saved is a penny earned," was popular after Benjamin Franklin coined it in hopes of teaching people how to "save for that rainy day." In this century we still hear that saying, but we probably say something closer to, "You won't have a pot to pee in," to warn people against reckless spending. "A bird in the hand is worth two in the bush," is another way forefathers taught our founders to appreciate what they had rather than gambling on chance. Now, a popular insurance company is using that image in a television commercial to promote services.

Sayings, brand names, and catch-words have a way of attaching to our energy and influencing our choices. Generic packaging is offered on most products, and while many of us will purchase some generics, most of us hold out for those things that we just have to have in the "original" form. And, even though we are told that many generically packaged products are produced at the same location as the original, we convince ourselves that a copy is not the same as the one we have always purchased (and, in some cases, as in some prescription medicines, this is true).

We let our choices become influenced by our emotions (the way we feel toward an item or issue). That is one of the reasons drug testing has to be done with a control group that either receives no treatment or placebos in lieu of the drug that is being tested. Placebos are not supposed to have a noticeable impact on a person's health since they are basically sugar pills, but our bodies do react to sug-

ar so some people may have weight gain, sluggish-
ness, euphoria, dizziness, or other pre-diabetic
symptoms.

Let's put those risks aside for the sake of our
discussion and focus on the mind-over-matter effect
some people have when taking placebos. Some
people believe in a source of healing so much that
they receive healing benefits even when nothing
new, other than that hope, has actually been added
to their systems.

So what could ramblings about what you say
(either internally or externally), how you refer to
names of products, drug testing, etc., have on you
and your heart health? They were all examples of
how we are inadvertently programmed to act or respond to various situations, and how our internal
"speak" is so innate we don't notice it, or suspect
how harmful it may be.

Following is a list of heart-related expressions that you may have attached to your energetic
being. Add any idioms you feel belong to the list
and pay close attention to any that resonate within
you (spark a feeling or emotion whether positive,
negative, or physical). Ensure you take time to im-
mediately journal your thoughts or feelings. Writing
down your feelings allows you to record where you
are at now for later review, and helps you to get

those feelings outside of Self (once you write it
down you start your healing process).

Broken hearted
My heart's broken

You've broken my
heart
Heartache

Heartburn
Lionhearted

Heart of gold

Heart of stone; ice

Coldhearted

Blow heart

Fainthearted
faint of heart

Half-hearted
Hard-hearted

Heart of stone

The heart wants what
the heart wants

Whole-hearted

Wearing your heart
on your sleeve

Guard your heart

Warm-hearted

Big-hearted

Heart as big as Texas

Heart reservations

Hole in his heart

Black heart

A piece of my heart

Room in my heart

A place in my heart

A part of my heart
died

Bleeding heart (liberal)

Brave heart

I feel it in my heart

A longing in my heart

A song in my heart

Made my heart sing

Light of my heart

My heart is fluttering

Closed hearted

Faint of heart

My heart goes out to you/them

With all of my heart

From the depths of my heart

Sound of heart

Heartbeat

My heart is racing

My heart stopped

My heart beats for you

I can hear your heartbeat

My heartfelt sympathy…

My heart went pitty pat

Hold you close in my heart

My heart is/was racing

You are my heart

He/She was my heart

For the sake of discussion, and to help show you a way to use this part of the process, let's say the cliché "big-hearted" triggered a reaction in me. Perhaps I could hear people using that term when describing me; maybe that is how I view myself; maybe I have had a diagnosis of "enlarged heart." Hearing or reading the phrase "big-hearted" may cause me to have good or bad feelings, but either way those feelings have an effect on me.

If I continue to experience these feelings I start to embrace (absorb) what is being said. What does that mean? It means I start to relay that information to my subconscious, which has no conscience. What does that mean? It means at a subconscious level I absorb the message that is being conveyed, and the subconscious has no way to interpret whether that message is good or bad for me, it simply works to serve me in an effort to help my wishes come true (its interpretation of my thoughts) so the Universe works to award me my big (or enlarged) heart.

For example, if I look in the mirror and tell myself "I look fat," my subconscious says "Okay, I'm fat," and it goes on a mission to help me realize that inner voice. Is this dangerous to me? Well, if it manifests as a bag or two of barbecue potato chips that I can work off with a bit more exercise, then "No." However, if I continue to let this inner voice have control, then I am destined to become what it tells me I am. No harm is done if I do not mind being fat, but when weight starts to affect my health I have to find a way to change that inner voice.

That is why it is so important for us to get in touch with the inner messages on which we operate. The hard thing is that we do not always know what the messages are. One thing for sure though is that if we let messages that are wrong for us stay in our subconscious, those messages will have an adverse effect on our bodies and overall health. Does that mean that everyone with extra weight has done this to themselves through self-talk? No, but that is a place to start if you are trying to lose the weight.

Of course you will have to recognize what these messages are, and since they can be virtually anything you let yourself think about or hear or read, the list is long and virtually endless. Here are some examples:

I have to be skinny to be popular.

I have to be rich to be successful.

I'm not as good as other people.

I'm not pretty.

I'm not a good person.

I can't date nice people; nice people aren't attracted to me.

I can't live with this disease.

My back is killing me.

This is suffocating me.

This is driving me insane.

I can't live without ….

My heart aches.

I can't take this anymore.

I have to do/be "x" to be loved/accepted/appreciated.

Fat people are stupid.

People who cuss are ignorant.

I'm going to win even if it kills me.

Other drivers are such assholes.

Customers can be such jerks.

I don't deserve "x" …

Whatever the inner voice is saying, it affects the choices you make, the way you feel, the efforts your unconscious self will go to in order to provide you what it thinks you desire, and your chances for happiness and health. The list provided was more of a depiction of negative self-speak.

But, what if you chose to intentionally implant positive messages? The subconscious has no conscience. It does not matter what the message is, your psyche is programmed to accept it and help you bring it into realization. Your mind actually creates matter. You can use that to your advantage when you want to create differences in your life.

I'm a great person.

I'm happy today.

I'm eating healthy food today.

I'm loveable.

I'm healthy.

I'm feeling better today.

I will smile today.

This does not rule my life.

I can change what I wish to change.

This is the best day ever.

Love wins out.

I choose to love you.

You're the best thing ever.

I can do this.

I can attract the things into my life that I need.

Many people call positive messages "mantras." A mantra is a phrase said over and over again to bring it into being. There are many books on the subject (of affirmations) that suggest writing down such phrases and putting them in places where they will be seen. That is a good idea, but the voices that get into the subconscious are more potent than a mantra pasted on your medicine cabinet. They are actually etched into your being.

The more stubborn, harmful voices are often those you hear from others—not because those voices are any more powerful than your own, but because we tend to believe others before we believe ourselves. Another aspect that makes outside voices so powerful is that they are usually repeated to a point where you learn to anticipate them.

In reality, you learn how to perform down to the standard the outside person(s) set. I say this because we are focusing on messages that need to be rerouted. Positive childhood messages can be just as influential to your wellbeing. If you are (were) consistently told that you can be anything you wish to be, it opens your mind (subconscious) to the hope of unlimited horizons.

We tend to trust other people before we trust our own inner voice because we spend up to two decades learning how to respect authority (or survive as the case may be), and that translates into listening to others. In a perfect world all of the authority figures we are subject to would be supportive and have only our best interests at heart. But that is not the world we live in, and what some people do in the best interests of others may not be what the persons in question need to develop healthy attitudes.

I suppose that is the bad news. But the good news is that we all come to the planet with purpose and many things to learn. I am of the opinion that we have specific goals in mind for our souls before we incarnate and we choose the parents with the most probability of helping us meet those challenges. (Probability because we all have free will and any member of the group we are born into has the right to quit or adjust the plan). This belief leads me to the theory that regardless of what we have been programmed to hear, think, believe (etc.), all of our experience goes into making each one of us an individual being.

Our exposures and experiences make us who we are. Or do they? Is it *what* we experience or *how* we integrate that experience that creates the beings we become? I suppose we also have choice in deciding between "what" or "how." If we choose "what" we experience we end up playing the role of Victim throughout our lives—we do not have to accept responsibility for ourselves or what we become because other people made us into who we are. Despite what happens, it happens *to* us and not because *of* us.

What do I mean? Suppose as a teenager we had a horrible home life; it came to a point that it was a matter of personal safety to escape, and as invincible head-strong youth we decided living on the streets was better than living with any stupid, abusive control-freak adult. We decide that all adults are corrupt or damaged and only want to harm us so we decide to hurt them first.

It becomes fine to steal from them or sell sex to them because we are using them. We feel we are in power but in reality we are victims. We have taken what has happened in our past life and made it into a part of any foreseeable future. Every time we "take advantage" of some new adult we are reasserting the fact that we are doing this because someone else did it to us.

Some might call this "an eye for an eye" logic, but it is Victim screaming out that it can't be right again until everyone guilty for its pain is punished (and that list is never extinguished, even if the original parties are punished). Victim's pain is not diminished as long as it lives in "what" happened (and relives that pain over and over again).

Should we choose "how" we integrate, we are taking our experiences from passive occurrences into the realm of active participation (even though it seems Victim is taking action, it is action based on occurrence and is passive because it is done in retaliation). In effect, we create who we are or who we wish to become. We do this when we select our mantras, when we choose to limit our exposure to negative people (or those we feel compromise our own best interests).

When you decide you want more out of life than the status quo you have allowed yourself to accept, and you open yourself to new ideas, you begin to create your own being. You allow your thoughts to change you. What do I mean? When we start to explore "how" something happened in our lives, how it came to be and how we were affected by it, we start a path of healing. True, we may never know the reasons horrible people were allowed into our lives, but if we can simply accept them as horrible people and move on, we can remove ourselves from their corrupt energy.

That doesn't mean that we have to accept what happened as wonderful, nor does it mean that we have to become friends with horrible people. In fact, cutting them out of our lives is recommended. Realizing "how" these situations came into being protects us from them happening again. We grow in wisdom, we learn that the world isn't always a safe place and we take measures to protect ourselves.

That same wounded teenager, once realizing "how" the situation happened (through corrupt adults) will seek out a way to eliminate corrupt adults from its energy field. Yes, the teen may be forced to endure the situation for a time, but it will scheme to find a way beyond the corruption and promise itself to never get close to that kind of corruption again. Whereas the teen living in "what" will immerse itself in like-energy (of corruption) while it seeks vengeance.

Homework:

1. Take some time to create a list of inner dialog you have allowed yourself to believe. It does not matter if you consider the entries to be negative or positive, but if you wish, you can create a separate list for each

2. List your health history annotating any inner thoughts you feel contributed

3. Keep your list of current/prior inner dialog for reflection (and additions) so you will have a record of past thought to compare with your health history; over the years, you may see comparisons/improvements

4. Explore occurrences in your past where you bogged down by "what" happened rather than working out "how" to move past it

5. Create a list of inner dialog you plan to adopt in order to improve your health situation.

6. Put a plan into action that helps you digest and then fully absorb this new way of thinking (e.g. pictures, mantras, friends, recordings, music, routines, prayer, color)

HEART STRINGS

*Everyone has a doctor
in him or her; we just
have to help it in its
work. The natural heal-
ing force within each
one of us is the greatest
force in getting well.*

Hippocrates

CHAPTER FIVE

Triggers

In Chapter Four we discussed harmful inner dialog.
When working with the heart chakra that is not
enough. We need to explore the triggers that exact
negative emotion. We all have them. We may have

cute expressions to disguise how much we are truly bothered by them, like, "He really knows how to push my buttons." But regardless, the buttons are being pushed, the emotions are gushing forward and eventually health is at risk.

How about the theory that venting feelings is positive? Is there danger to Type A people who consistently yell (when under pressure)? What about the heart attacks we see on television where someone turns red like an erupting volcano, yells and then keels over?

People who consistently yell have anger and control issues. Does that mean they are at risk for heart attack? That depends on if the anger is internalized or not. Drill instructors yell and find countless things to comment about, but they have a mission to mold strong military people. If the anger is simply a front then there probably is not danger to the body. You have probably met someone who is consistently yelling regardless of apparent mood—it is simply that person's nature to do so.

If the anger is triggered from somewhere inside, then the person does run a risk. What does that mean? If the yelling person has always yelled and it has become a part of the character, there may not be as much risk—that is simply an angry, manipulative or self-absorbed person that may benefit from having some of his own medicine. If the anger comes in spurts and is driven by some kind of event (trigger), then it is more of an eruption, which is pressure on the entire system, and something has to blow. In most cases it is the temper expressed in some way that aims to destroy everything in its path. But that same temper could be rerouted into less volatile "steam vents" that aim to gently ease the pressure.

You have probably heard some of the more popular venting advice through the years: count to ten before you say anything; take three deep breaths before you react; go to the gym and work it out; get a miniature Zen garden and rake the sand; listen to water; listen to calming classical music; laugh, even when you do not feel like laughing. All good approaches to diffusing anger as long as you ensure the emotion is rerouted and not simply capped off. If your answer is to bottle up the anger and not express it you run just as much risk, if not more, to heart health.

No one is going to be able to avoid the emotion of anger, it has to exist for there to be joy, otherwise there would be no way to measure happiness. People, especially energy workers, who try to avoid anger are not serving their own greater good. Anger exists. It is best to acknowledge anger, embrace it and find productive ways to use it rather than to decide anger will not be a part of your life.

People choosing the avoidance path run as much risk to heart health as the erupting people because both are merely storing up rage that the body will eventually have to discharge. The expression "blow a gasket" comes to mind.

It is very important for you to know what triggers your anger. Start a list, and once you have that list, start working on ways to either eradicate those triggers or short fuse them. Avoiding anger-provoking situations may not be possible, but you are a being of choice and you can choose not to let anger rule your life.

To help get you started I will share some of my anger triggers: customer service people who have no concept of what customer service is; tele-marketers, regardless of when they call; bad or un-safe drivers; my cat who yowls for food as I am dishing out the wet food—every day, twice a day.

Knowing your triggers is part of the battle, diffusing the triggers is quite another thing. Lacka-daisical customer service people can be handled. Your goal is to get the service you desire. Make it a game, use your cunning, do everything except make it personal. Once it becomes personal you own the problem of the others' errant behavior. You will be the one storing up the bad energy from the confron-tation while the other person may not give the encounter another thought. Once it becomes personal you start to engage anger and it could result in flared tempers which serves no one, even if you have had to repeat the same information 10 times because you got disconnected 5 times.

Telemarketers are a different issue altogether. With customer service people you usually can prepare for the encounter, telemarketers ambush you. You are usually in the safety of your own home, doing something intimate to your being (even if it is paying bills), and the stranger intrudes on your peace to offer you something you do not need or want. It is aggravating—or is it?

My sister and brother-in-law actually talk with the people, listen to the spiel, and politely decline whatever the offer is. It amazes me that they can be so patient and kind, when they are usually in a flurry of chaos managing homework, dinner, chores and myriad miscellaneous household duties required by a young and growing family. I tend to express my displeasure for the interruption, threaten the poor person with "no call list" violation litigation, and end with a loud slam of the phone (I still have one that can be slammed down; the end-talk button ones do not satisfy my rage).

Sometimes I do not speak; I merely slam the phone down once I know it is an annoying call. I do have to admit though that the energy of the exchange sets badly with me. I dwell on the call and my reaction to it several hours after the encounter. The telemarketer may or may not dwell on people's reactions—one would have to have a dismissive personality to survive long in such a job. My sister probably has the right idea—treat others as you would like to be treated, even if you are busy or completely uninterested in what they have to say. You decide (if this is a trigger for you).

There is no rational way to describe the relationship I have with my older cat. He is a cat-cat—wants attention on his own terms, is not very affectionate, and if he does not get his way he will find a way to let me know. He can regurgitate at will and ensures his efforts are strategically placed in well trodden, yet unobserved, areas. He insists on being fed wet food morning and night, even though he has dry food continuously available. He also gets bored with the wet food and has to have something different everyday as long as it is not fish, except for tuna, which he prefers mixed with chicken or egg, unless he is sharing my people tuna. In other words, he is a picky, persnickety cat.

I tolerate these quirks in his character; after all, he is elderly for a cat and deserves a certain amount of consideration. The one thing that "drives me up the wall" is his yowling. It starts the nanosecond he sees the catfood can in my hand and does not stop until the bowl is placed in front of him, which is several minutes because it has to be cleaned. I feel like he is nagging me and let's just say it does not set well with me. I have tried so many things to divert my attention or to help me ignore the cat's behavior, but must admit that typically I end up yelling right back at him and making all kinds of aimless threats (which are energetically harmful).

Of course I have explored my past relationships to see what behaviors the cat is mirroring back to me. I have used the cat as a teacher to help me learn more patience. I have tried to talk back to him in similar cat language (of which I am not the least fluent). Singing, cajoling, laughing, I have tried it all. I simply have a cat that has a horribly annoying habit, if I choose it to be annoying, and that is the truth of the matter. Some days I handle the cat better than others; some days the anger wins.

Life is not always neat and nice. We simply have to find ways to make it past the bumps without disturbing our inner peace. (Yeah, right! Try maintaining inner peace with a yowling cat at your heals).

There is a need here to bring up the topic of the "loud family." Some families are quiet, polite and well mannered. Other families reside at the other end of that spectrum—loud, brusque and going out of the way to embarrass others with bodily sounds. To those on the outside it seems as if these people are always arguing. Outsiders rarely understand that "bickering" is simply the language of the clan, and volume is the way one is heard. What is amazing (to outsiders if they realize it), is that these people are not upset with each other. They do not even feel that they are arguing and are amazed when outsiders react to what they are saying.

Psychologists will tell you that throwing pots and pans is okay as long as both partners accept that as a form of expression. To relate this to the above example, it becomes trouble in a relationship if one partner is closed and reserved, and the other is loud and expressive. If the expressive partner launches an object, the reserved partner feels it is a personal attack and charges the other with abuse. That was merely an example, I am not condoning cookware wars, but the same applies for verbalization. Yelling is not bad or good, judgment rests with the audience.

I am typically a quiet person. I can go for days without uttering a word (except around cat feeding time, or if a telemarketer calls). But when I am around others I give myself permission to become whatever feels best. If I am excited, I tend to be loud. I remember my brother inviting me to use my "inside voice" during one of our family visits (I only wish I could remember what we were doing).

My daughter and I have a history of loud discussions that end up with each of us trying to get our own points across. An outsider would call this arguing, and it is to a point, but within our inner circle it is a way of preserving our cherished memories. My sister-in-law once told me that it takes two to argue, so it was clear that she was laying the burden for remedying this behavior on my doorstep. It was also clear that she did not condone excessive emotion in her family. I learned a lot from her, and used her technique of not playing along with my daughter's need to argue when it served me (the family).

With that said, it is also important for me to honor my daughter's personality. She expresses herself in a bold, non-apologetic manner that is innate to her being. I do not remember being that type of person, but I am more apt to yell up the stairs than I am to quietly go up and tell someone they are needed. I have also been called stubborn and bull-headed when I feel something should be a certain way, or know that I am right about something (even after I am shown how wrong I am). My daughter no-doubt picked up on these personality quirks and added them to her arsenal by ways of defense if not offense.

We have also noticed that she behaves differently when we are around family members than she does when we are one-on-one. We have a pleasant, quiet relationship when we are alone. Exposed to family she somehow feels the need to gain their blessing and seems to do it by defacing my credibility with family members. It may have been because she spent so much time with my mother that she felt more like a competitive sibling at times than like a loved and accepted daughter.

We truly do not know, but discussing the issues has helped us diffuse it a bit. Not that there was anything wrong to begin with, but because I want her to be seen as the sweet person she can be by other family members. Of course her grandparents always love her unconditionally, as does the rest of the family (in small doses at times). I can say this now that she is an adult with a child quickly approaching the teen years.

I have mellowed with age, and with education, but I do remember feeling agitated, unappreciated and basically invalidated when my daughter struggled through her teen years. Civility was not our forte at that time, but there is life after teen (for all concerned).

What do you do if you are the only quiet

person in a very loud family? You learn to cope and seek out peaceful sanctuaries as you can. It may be easier for you to blend in than it is for the one loud person in a very quiet family. Our families are provided to us as a way of familiarizing us with the workings of the world—we cannot expect everyone within a family to exhibit cloned behavior. It is the vast differences that help us perform better in society; a part of us knows what to anticipate from strangers, which provides us with a cushion as we go out into the world.

So what do triggers and the expressive differences in people around us have to do with personal heart health? Our vascular system is a closed one, it relays on its own internal pressure to keep and maintain a steady flow. Eruptions of anger, or repressing and internalizing anger, put pressure on this very delicate system. That internal pressure can also be something as simple as pushing yourself to accomplish more when your body is trying to tell you it's tired and needs to rest.

It is important for you to know what "sets you off." Occasional spurts of this kind of pressure are fine in youth, but as you age you have built up quite a history of these spurts, and like a dormant volcano that vents steam in an effort to release build-up, you are in danger of that underlying pressure that threatens to cause a major eruption. Once you identify problem areas, make efforts to nullify them (my adolescent niece loves to feed my cat—I emphatically encourage her kitty relationship).

Homework:

1. Make a list of your triggers. It may help for you to picture yourself in multiple situations
2. If your list had less than 20 items on it, carry your notebook around with you for a week or more so you can jot down things that get you steamed as they happen
3. Once you have your list, look for similarities in what starts the pot to boil and group your trigger events if you can; note that some triggers can be environmental or nutritional in nature (e.g. low blood sugar, over-caffeination; fear of storms)
4. Make another list of the things you (can) do to help you diffuse the event; remember that anger is not evil, it is fine to have anger, but you do not want to have eye-popping, vein swelling, face reddening, cat kicking explosions that cause strain on your vascular system and heart

HEART STRINGS

*Prayer indeed is good, but while
calling on the gods
A man should himself lend
a hand.*

Hippocrates

CHAPTER SIX

Heart Related

There are peripheral physical ailments associated with heart dis-ease that can occur throughout the body rather than strictly within the heart muscle. Since they are energetically (and physically) tied to heart health it is important for us to discuss them and their chakral connections.

STROKES

Strokes (Ischemic, Hemorrhagic), aneurysm,

cerebrovascular accident (blood clots), are being grouped into the 6th chakra but also have ties to the 1st chakra. The 6th chakra is where "thought" is energetically managed. So could a person think a stroke away? After all, we have been discussing mind over matter.

That is not how to use the knowledge of what lives in a particular chakra. It is more accurate to review what is listed as "living" within a chakra. Logic and rationalization are maintained in the 6th chakra, but a stroke can have many causes. Thinking alone (probably) cannot stop a stroke, but if you are at risk for stroke or recovering from stroke, it may help to review *how* you think, and *what* you think.

It is important to determine what your thoughts have been. Changing your thoughts, especially ones steeped in anger or ones on a continuous worry loop, may help to decrease vascular stress. Humor is especially helpful in changing thoughts. It is almost impossible to be angry or actively worried when you are laughing.

Blood clots can actually occur anyplace in the body so they are more of a 1st chakra (vascular) issue. If you have clots (e.g. post surgical) it does not mean they are a result of external family problems (to pick one example from what the 1st Chakra holds). In fact, the clots may have nothing to do with your energy management system.

Sometimes physical issues are purely physical in nature and not incumbent to any emotional or spiritual energy. Some clots are a result of surgery or injury. Could those be attached to some kind of energetic imbalance? Yes, but they could just as easily be physical in nature. Ancestry in the form of genetic heritage may have predisposed you toward experiencing blood clots but may have nothing to do with you actually having a clot. Sometimes an illness is simply an illness and asking "Why?" does not get you answers.

But, if you are earnest in your quest to unravel physical ailments and there is an energetic connection, knowing yourself and being open to exploring your thoughts is a step forward in providing you with answers. Vascular issues can occur when outside pressures are greater on your system than the internal pressure you are able to maintain. Or, you could put more pressure (internally) onto yourself than outside influences expect. Either way there is an imbalance. What do I mean? Think of the pressure on your vascular system as being two people arm wrestling. The players would have to be equal in strength to maintain the contest; as soon as one player over-exerts the other, the contest is over—one player wins, the other collapses.

We all need to be able to stand up for ourselves, but in reality learning how to exert Self is a challenge some of us are contracted to learn. What does that mean? We spend our lives learning. What we learn is largely up to each one of us, but some things are necessary in order for us to fulfill our life journey. You may be contracted to learn how to assert yourself.

It is not my desire to get into a debate over predetermination, fate or other theoretical issues. There are theorists who believe we do not come to the planet to learn (lessons). It is my belief that we all come to the planet with an agreement, contract if you will, with God to accomplish certain things. Whether or not we comply with the terms of the contract is up to each one of us, and we are allowed to renegotiate points of the contract.

But, major experiences must be endured in order for us to accomplish the goals that we each set for ourselves before we incarnate. So, when we start to doubt our purpose for being here, or ask God to give us some kind of sign to let us know what our purpose is, we are actually asking to review the contract we originated.

Some of us do make contracts to further medical research by letting ourselves become conduits of illness. It takes a brave and evolved soul to sacrifice a life to forward medical knowledge. Some of us contract illness in order to heal (family) relationships. Some of us contract illness to pay back some karmic debt contracted in this life or a past-life.

How would you know if you have a contract to have an illness (traumatic experience) or if you are simply ill? Contracted illness (or traumatic experience) may simply seem to make sense at some deep, inner level. Proof is something you will never have; you will have to have faith in the peace of mind you receive when answers are received. What do I mean? If you pray about your situation, the Universe will hear you, answer you, and grant you peace. You will also know if there are more things you need to explore. Remember, Sixth Chakra holds your God connection that is why prayer is something to explore, especially with Sixth Chakra issues.

Believing in contracts, purpose, karma, etc., is a leap of faith. We all have some kind of belief system. You do not have to ascribe to mine; you simply have to explore what your beliefs are, then you will better know how to handle Sixth Chakra energy issues. Just remember, even if you lean toward atheism, humans naturally seek out some power greater than Self to believe in. Agnostics may try to deny this need, but perhaps they are serving a path that will help others make spiritual decisions. One might also say that choosing not to believe is in itself "belief."

Do you have to believe in a higher power to do energy work? If you believe healing is done with God energy, then believing in God would be desirable. But, you can take the scientific approach and call the energy "electricity." You can do research into Kirlian photography, crystal growing, light and sound effects on the human body, copper bracelets, magnets, static electricity, etc.—there is plenty of scientific data on the body's energetic emanations.

If you or a loved one has already experienced a stroke there are many alternative medicine disciplines you may wish to explore to help restore function to the body. Effectiveness will depend upon the damage done to the brain. If the damage is primarily to nerves, energy work may be helpful. Massage, chiropractic intervention, acupuncture, aromatherapy, Reiki, Pranic Healing, sound therapy, image therapy, meditation, and chakra exploration are but a few avenues available to you. There may be help received through acts of forgiveness and exploration of how control (judgement, external stressors, etc.) issues may have contributed to the vascular issues.

It is important to first determine the cause of

the stroke—whether it was from a blockage (fear to move forward, difficulty letting go); clot (avoidance of stressful issues, unresolved stress issues, temporary Band-Aids on problems); or aneurysm (continued grating of same old issues, feeling helpless to avoid/remedy the cause of stress).

Once you determine what the cause was, and where it was located, you can explore the symbolism the Universe is providing you in unraveling the energetics associated with your situation. If you are doing this for a loved one you may have to interpret the symbols from the loved one's point of view, but in my experience the Universe speaks to each of us in our own language. What does that mean? You will only have to interpret what the symbols mean to you and then apply them to your loved one.

By way of example, let's say a woman had a blood clot as a result of giving birth. The clot was unnoticed until she started exhibiting paralysis and there was real danger of the clot moving and causing stroke or worse. That is all we need to know to start investigating Second Chakra issues. Was she inordinately concerned with becoming a mother? Is she afraid she will not be a good parent? Has she bonded with the child? Was the child taken from her against her wishes or her conscience? Now that she has the child is she concerned about her way forward? Is she financially challenged? Is she afraid she will not be able to provide the values needed to raise a successful child? Is she depressed over not being given the chance to raise the child?

Once you ask the questions, and have tentative answers, you have a place to start looking for avenues of (energetic) healing.

Exploring the answers to the questions you come up with that apply to your unique situation is a start to understanding the energetic connections you or your loved one has with the physical ailment at hand. Will that exploration automatically resolve all of the physical issues? Perhaps not. The ailment may still require surgery, medication or physical therapy, but working with the energetics behind the ailment will greatly aid in recovery and prevention of further episodes. Is there a guarantee that energy work will alleviate the problem? No, no more so than any medical procedure can guarantee. The human body and the energetic body are mysteries we can only hope to explore.

LUNGS

There are differences between Eastern and Western philosophies on many fronts so why should energy placement opinions be any exception? In Western philosophy grief is managed in the heart; in

Eastern philosophy grief lives in the lungs. Why bring that up here since this is a book primarily focused on a Western audience? I bring it up because while we are primarily discussing heart-related illness, the Fourth Chakra includes the lungs, so the energies of the chakra apply to both heart and lungs.

Grief can become an entity of its own. When people experience loss, whether expected or traumatic, there is no way of knowing how long grief will take up residence. To a degree, a significant emotional event never really leaves our energy field. We are complex creatures and can compartmentalize our emotions, which can be helpful and harmful.

It is better to process emotion, but if processed emotions still reside within us, where do they live? In the case of grief, the residual processed grief is also compartmentalized within the heart chakra. But how do we know how many times we can safely access the storage facility? If something is truly processed, why would we drag it all out again, and what would be left to drag out? If something were hidden away, how long can it stay until we must process it? If we keep processing past events are we merely feeding them (energy we need for current issues) thereby keeping them tethered to us? How, if ever, do we rid ourselves of the past so we have enough energy to live comfortably in our present?

We do not choose who (or what) to grieve over. Sometimes we have no choice. Of course there are the obvious people (parents, spouses, children, best friends, lovers), but sometimes we do not know how important people are to us until they are gone. Celebrities fall into this category (the world still mourns Michael Jackson), but there are also events that we grieve (Sep 11, 2001; assassinations; war crimes; cult killings; school shootings; Superbowl losses, etc.).

Grief is normal for humans, and healthy. There are books written to help us through the grieving process and to help us aid others through the process. Academics have even broken the process down into stages. We are all familiar with grief. So why should I bring it up?

Our systems can handle emotion, but there is a limit to how much of a negative emotion we can safely handle before that emotion starts to deplete our reserves. Before I go further, I should acknowledge fellow energy workers who may want to argue that there are no negative or positive emotions, emotions simply "are." I feel that argument has merit, so for sake of our discussion I will define negative emotions as "any emotions that deplete our energy reserves."

What do I mean? The emotion itself is neither positive nor negative, it is simply provided to us as a vehicle to express our being. But, sometimes we get stuck within the process of expression and we cannot quite let go. If we are allowed to remain stuck while processing grief we will actually start grieving grief instead of the person or event that initially brought us into the abyss.

For the sake of discussion let's say that there are positive and negative emotions, with the difference being ones that feed us and ones that deplete us. But if I were to ask you to make a list, it would be harder to tell if an emotion is depleting you than it would be to make a list of negative emotions.

What do I mean? Let's take the emotion of love. Love would probably be put on the "positive" emotion list. But what if someone becomes obsessed with another person to the point of smothering, controlling, or stalking? The defense for those actions will be "love" but obsession is an emotion within itself (that could belong in any chakra depending on the subject of the obsession). The parent that controls a child to the point of abuse will say it is done out of love. We selectively choose our labels for our actions, which makes compiling a positive and negative list of emotions difficult at best.

But what of the emotion of hate; is hate ever

used in a positive way? Our "hatred" of oppression drove us to explore new countries, fight for civil rights and oppose genocide. Hate can stir us into action, but if used in a negative way it can drain us of energy needed to run the body. It will not happen overnight, but eventually the chakra's reserves will be depleted and the body will suffer. Like any other emotion, hate in itself is neutral. It is how we choose to employ emotion that makes it positive or negative—innocent or harmful.

The Forth Chakra, more than others, is sensitized toward pent up emotion. The Forth Chakra acts as a gateway between the lower chakras (which are about "me" support), and the upper chakras, which connect us to more altruistic energies. Before we can take on any cause we must obtain Heart Chakra approval. "Taking it to heart" is the mantra for this vote of approval for if our hearts are not in what we do our projects will fizzle.

Thinking about lungs is important also because they are our vehicles for releasing used up energy. No-doubt you have been told to take a deep breath and release it to help your system back to a state of calm. "Out with the old (air, energy) and in with the new."

What if you could not release pent up energies? What if a deep breath was something you could not take because your lungs were filled with fluid? "Drowning in my tears" is the mantra for the grief the lungs hold. Living in perpetual grief is like slowly drowning (in grief).

There is a reason that "drowning in my sorrow" is an expression that has stood the test of time. The saying originally represented tears of sorrow but through the years has come to mean attempting to drown sorrow in alcohol (hence the change of the saying to "drowning my sorrow"). The symbolic parallels between crying toxic amounts of tears and imbibing toxic liquids are interesting, but many people who chronically grieve do not drink alcohol. Charles Dickens captured chronic grief through the character of Miss Havisham in his classic novel, Great Expectations.

One diagnosis for fluid in the lungs is pneumonia—does that mean if you get pneumonia that you have so much grief that you are drowning? No. But that is certainly an area to explore if you have repeated bouts with pneumonia. Processing grief can make you more susceptible to pneumonia, colds, bronchitis and other illnesses resulting in congestion or weakness to the lungs or air passages. If you are actively processing grief ensure you boost your immune system the same way you would arm yourself against a cold.

Emphysema is the inability to breathe due to damaged lung tissue usually caused by outside sources (cigarette smoke, coal dust, asbestos, fiberglass, etc.). Environment can certainly be a contributor to illness, but if you have an environmental exposure does it cancel your need to explore an emotional contributor to the condition? No, because you need to explore what led you to choose that form of exposure.

What do I mean? You did not have to smoke, or live in a mining community or choose the job that exposed you to the danger. Why did you? Was it a contract you made prior to incarnating? If so, explore what you have learned and what you have yet to experience to help you fulfill your journey. [And, "No," no one can tell you what you have to experience; there are no shortcuts, only you will know when you have completed your contract. With that said, energy workers can tell if there is any energy left in a contract, but I do not advise you to try and cheat—if you are through with a contract you will feel "complete."]

Whatever lung diseases you are experiencing, look at your emotional involvement in the process. In particular, look at your relationship to grief, being sure you do not limit yourself to the grief surrounding loss of life. There are many more types of grief and one of them may be what is draining your energy (e.g. loss of job; loss of career opportunity; loss of a car; loss of a love; best friend moving away; losing a deal; loss of home/belongings; loss of health; old issues you cannot seem to escape, etc.). Once you know what your relationship to grief is, with some work you can learn how to bring joy back into your life.

Humans are gregarious creatures. We require social interaction to live healthy, balanced lives. Of course there are exceptions and you may be able to name a hermit or recluse that functions well completely cut off from society. But the typical diagnosis for antisocial people is "sociopath" which involves a complete lack of conscience toward fellow humans (the ability to kill and maim with no guilt or remorse). There are also mental illnesses that disable some people from actively integrating social skills, but as a norm we are social creatures.

We form attachments with other humans. We call people "loved ones" to label our special groups, and we make our "lists" of people who offend. Once someone is in our intimate group it does not matter how far he moves away or how long he stays gone, that person is almost always held dear. If something devastating happened to dissolve the relationship, that person will still be remembered (to some degree). In fact, it is usually the devastating endings we remember when recalling old loves. We might grieve over that kind of lost love, more than one that simply dissolved amicably.

KIDNEYS, ADRENALS

Reno vascular Hypertension and Renal Artery Stenosis are both illnesses on the periphery of heart dis-ease, as they are complications suffered because of heart related illness. The 2nd Chakra is looked to for the energetic support of the renals and kidneys, but this is also a vascular situation, so the 1st Chakra may be engaged.

Does this mean that renal compromise is related to relationships? Did those failed romances lead you to the predicament that you are in now? That depends. Yes, the 2nd Chakra is the energy center for personal relationships, but your energy drain may have nothing to do with relationships. There are many other energies in the chakra that may have ties to your situation. You are the best judge of which ones to explore. Same thing goes for the failed romances. But, if you still dwell over lost loves years after you have moved on, especially if you are in another relationship now, this would be something to seriously explore.

The dynamics of how we feel toward another person can overrun our ability to do what is best for ourselves. There are times when we fall in love with a person who simply cannot love us in return. Other times we are the ones with the admirer we cannot abide. Denying another person can be as draining on our chakral system as longing for someone we cannot have. Our systems can handle most of this give and take of energy exchange for a while, but in a perfect world we eventually find that "one" person and settle down, which is supposed to balance out the energy.

What if we are exceptions to the norm and continue to have failed relationships decades past our friends who married in high school? It would be wise to ensure we are not losing energy to those "old news" people; and, that we have learned something through the years about the types of partners we simply cannot tolerate. If we are still attracted to the same old type of wrong person after all of these years then why are we surprised that our relationships keep failing? Why, too, are we surprised that we have drainage causing health problems in the chakra managing relationship energy?

If you feel your problems may rest in this area, you may want to consider celibacy until you can bring your energy back into alignment. If that path seems too drastic to you, dig deep into the relationships you have had. Find the similarities and the differences between the people you have been involved with. Study the relationships that you ended and that were ended for you. Determine which ones you dwell on the most. If you have forgiveness issues to process then do your best to resolve that part of the equation. Do what you must do to stop the lost love movie loop you have playing in your mind, and stop bleeding energy that you need to bring this part of your body back to balance.

The same advice goes for whatever energy of the second chakra you feel has caused the drain in your system. If you feel your kidneys have been compromised you can have your doctor do blood work to ensure you don't have physical problems that need to be addressed. If your problem is with the adrenals you may have to address your issues with (the emotions of) stress; you can't make everything urgent, scary or an emergency. Your body needs some down time to relax, and not just during sleep; your mind also needs some time to relax (while it is conscious) and daydream.

Homework:

1. Follow the suggestions under the heading that most applies to your situation
2. Be sure to explore other chakras and physical systems if you have situations we have not covered here; do not be afraid to use your own intuition to arrive at helpful ways to bring yourself back to balance
3. If you have a situation not covered here, write it into your notebook and break it down into chakras so you can make a plan on how to explore the (stored) emotions that may have contributed

*Every tomorrow has two handles. We can take hold
of it with the handle of anxiety or the handle of
faith.*

Henry Ward Beecher

CHAPTER SEVEN

Energy Work Sampler

We have done a lot of talking about energy
and energy work. There are a variety of re-
sources you can find to further your study in
areas that peak your interest, but I would
feel remiss if I did not provide you with a

peek into areas that might attract you on your path toward better heart health and emotional balance.

Music

Music therapy is a broad area with many facets you can explore that can improve chakra health. Each chakra radiates to a specific musical note and phonetic sound. A simple way to balance chakras is to sing out loud, but it must be a song that covers more than one octave and has a variety of vowel sounds. I find songs from the 1960s to the 1980s (or older 'do-wap' songs) are the best. I personally sing to the 1961 version of, "The Lion Sleeps Tonight" by the Tokens.

If you want to do more you can try crystal bowls, chanting, flutes, or simply playing music you find soothing. Classical music is very conducive toward establishing a balance in the energy of your home or place of meditation. Drumming is used in many cultures but it is primarily to assist achievement of a trance state, which serves to harmonize the body with vibrations of the earth.

Color

Colors vibrate at specific energies. You scientists will appreciate the fact that the only way we can see color is because it travels on a certain wavelength. Each chakra is also designated by a color (but do not get dismayed if sources do not agree on each color, decide for yourself). In a simple breakdown accepted by a majority of energy-related texts, the First Chakra is red; Second Chakra is orange; Third Chakra is yellow; Forth Chakra is pink or green; Fifth Chakra is blue (turquoise, aqua, topaz); Sixth Chakra is purple.

There are many ways to use color to facilitate chakra health. You can pay more attention to the colors that you choose to wear or that comfort you. The colors that you use to decorate your home will give you hints into what chakras you are comfortable with, or working on. Painting your walls bright yellow could mean you are at home with your ego, or you are working on self-esteem issues. Your home is also your fortress. You tend to decorate it in colors that soothe you or remind you of your contracts. You will know at some internal level why you have been attracted to the colors you love—do not worry about picking apart every decision you make, just know at some level you are helping yourself feel safe and protected.

Many people wear clothing in colors that help protect them or remind them of the chakra energies they are working on, confronting or processing in that moment. That is also a reason that some energy workers prefer to wear black—it is soothing because it absorbs the energy of color and doesn't fight for a prominent place; it is a quiet color (even though many consider it dramatic, and in some cases evocative).

Gemstones

Gemstones can help you focus on chakras you are working on, concerned about, or feel might be challenged. Advanced levels of Pranic Healing teach the use of gemstones and crystals for healing and energy focusing. Since the actual use of gemstones is an advanced technique, I only encourage you to use gemstones to help your mind focus on the issues concerning you. You would not need to use gemstones as a focus reminder; the colors you are wear would work just as well.

One thing you will have to keep in mind is that crystals (gemstones) have simple intelligence—they pick up psychic imprints from anyone touching them. You will have to learn how to clean your crystals and protect them from grabby people. If you are consecrating your crystals to perform protective tasks for you, you will have to take care to honor and respect them. If you do not know how to work with crystals find someone who can teach you or bless/instruct them for you. Beware that everyone working in a metaphysical shop is not proficient in all of the nuances of the items sold. Ask for a reference so you can learn the technique for yourself, or ask about the energy healing modalities in which they are certified.

Gemstones you can use in the chakras we have discussed are: First Chakra, ruby or garnet, the redder the better; Second Chakra, Madera citrine, amber (though some will argue that is a resin, not a gemstone); Third Chakra, yellow citrine, canary diamond; Fourth Chakra, pink tourmaline, pink diamond, rose quartz, peridot, emerald (but most use a lighter shade of green than emeralds); Fifth Chakra, blue topaz (but since it is a radiated stone some advise against it for healing purposes), aqua marine (but it is better for psychic connection than for healing); turquoise (but it is a stone and not a gemstone so the energy is more dense), moonstone; Sixth Chakra, amethyst.

Cleopatra and her priests used Russian amber to induce psychic awareness, but amber is a resin and not a stone, so it will not feel or react the same as a gemstone. There are several different colors of amber that can be used for healing if you choose. Many references will say amber (orange) is the "gemstone" for the second chakra. The Second Chakra is problematic in that there are not many naturally colored orange gemstones. If you are attracted to a lab-created stone then use it. Lab-created stones have the same molecular composition as natural gemstones but some healers feel their vibrations are not as strong, which will not matter since you are not using the stone for healing. If you find a rock (many varieties do have orange veins), then use that. For your purposes of using the gemstones for focus, you can take broader liberties with your choices.

Pranic Healing teaches that only rose

quartz or white quartz should be worn over
the heart chakra. This would be good to
keep in mind if you are experiencing heart-
related problems, especially if you wear a lot
of natural jewelry. Rhodilite has an extremely strong vibration especially in the larger
stones. Pay close attention to how your body
feels when you are wearing natural pieces. If
you feel dizzy, drained, or on edge you may
need to put those pieces aside until your
chakra health is better. Regardless of chakra
strength, some stones may simply not set
well with you. Best to know that before investing in them.

If you love jewelry, or simply feel
better adorning yourself, research objects
worn around the world to see if you, through
a past-life, are attracted to them. Pearls,
jade, shells, bone, feathers, herbs are just a
few examples of items that are worn for protective or energetic purposes.

If you are fond of crystals, they are
used in many forms of energy healing (to
include Feng Shui), but take time to do your
research. Crystals require care and can
overwhelm the energy in a space if you are
not careful. Several sources recommend
keeping them out of your bedroom especial-

ly if you have trouble sleeping.

Kinetic Energy

We have established the fact that everything radiates energy. Some people are sensitive to energetic vibrations. You can research auras to learn more about the energy field surrounding every human. An aura is basically an invisible (to most eyes) sack of energy surrounding each of us like a bubble. If you can see auras, you may see them as waves, gray/white/black fog-like puffs, or full-blown color palates.

According to what sources you read, there may be differences in how many layers an aura has (how many bubbles encase us), or what they are named—do not dwell on that, find what makes sense to you and start there. The important thing is to know that you can probably learn how to feel auras if you work at it. Since that is energy you are already used to it will be easier and more familiar for you to sense.

A crucial first step is to learn to respect energy. There are people working in energy fields that do not take precautions to dispose of discarded energy properly and it

ends up returning to the individual or finding another host. Reading this book does not
qualify you to move energy or experiment
on other people unless you are using them as
simple models that you can try to "feel."
Should you want to go beyond that you must
seek further training.

It will be easier to start if you do
some simple exercises to warm up your
hands. The more the blood flow to them the
easier it is to make kinetic connections. As
you practice you may eventually find it un-
necessary to prepare your hands. Put your
hands up in front of you palms out and flex
your fingers as if you are squeezing a ball of
air five to ten times. Then clench your hands
together with fingers interlocking and do
about a dozen squeeze-and-release repeti-
tions. You will know when you have done
enough to start feeling energy in your hands,
and the more you practice using kinetic energy, the fewer the required squeezes. You
can also shake your hands a few times or
squeeze your hands together in a tight self-
handshake to warm up.

Before you start it may help you to
have an idea of what to expect when feeling
energy. Bear in mind that it is not the same

for everyone, you may feel buzzing, prickles, itching, temperature changes, etc., but the most common thing to feel when merely sensing a kinetic connection is a magnetic pull. If you have two magnets around the house (that attract each other and stick together) put them together and pull them apart noticing how the "pull" feels. That energy of "attraction" is what you will feel in your hands.

Warm up your hands and then put them in front of you palms together (just like the magnets). Slowly move your hands apart one to three inches, and then back together. Repeat this motion until you can feel the energy pulsing between your hands. When you can comfortably feel the energy, move your hands further apart from each other. Work at this (not all at one time) until you can feel the energy between your hands when they are 12 to 18 inches apart.

Once you can feel your own energy at that distance you are ready to practice with a partner. Most sources agree that a standard personal aura is a distance of about three feet from the person emanating it (not the same as the 3-inch energy aura that surrounds you). Since chakras also emanate cones of energy (within your aura), we must ensure that we do not disturb them, or confuse them with the auric field.

Most Chakra energy is sent out from a person's chest and back, so it is best for beginners to practice feeling auras on the sides of people. Stand a foot or two away from your model, face to face or face to back, but a bit to the side so you can push your hand into the person's aura. You will be making a full-armed sweeping motion to locate the auric border emanating from your model's side. With your extended arm about shoulder height, move it toward the model's side until you feel resistance.

There are several layers to the aura. One is about three inches from the body. This one is not recommended for beginners to start with (but this is the one most people can see). The easiest aura to feel is the one about three feet away, but stronger auras can be 5 to 6 feet away so you need to make sure you allow enough distance for your sweep to pick up the border.

For some energy workers and spiritual leaders the aura is so subtle and so large that it emanates multiple feet. A person like that would have to concentrate in order to allow you to feel the immediate energy field. Actually we all have an auric field beyond the 3-foot zone, but why make this any more confusing than it needs to be?

You are working toward feeling the outside border of the personal aura. The entire zone is pulsating with energy, but the border will be more concentrated. You will feel a definite resistance. Practice until you are sure you can feel it on your partner and then try working with a new model to validate your new-found talent. If your teacher suggests starting with the 3-inch aura, then start there; there are no hard and fast rules for beginners, the goal is to feel…anything energetic.

Once you are confident you can feel aura energy you can try experimenting with inanimate objects. Try feeling the difference between colors, or go out in the yard and see if there is a difference between how a rock and a tree feel. Surely you will find plenty of things to practice on once you get started.

One thing I use kinetic energy for is to help me select books at the store. Sometimes the number of books on a certain topic is overwhelming; at other times I am trying to select the perfect gift for a friend. I put my intention into my thought and ask the Universe to help show me the book that would be best to help me reach my greater good (or the greater good of the person I am shopping for). I then run the palm of my hand past the books on the shelf and wait for the magnetic attraction to draw me to my book. It has never failed.

It would be wise to take notes on what you feel when you sense an energetic connection, or get an intuitive signal, because this is how the Universe communicates with you. Just remember that you are simply feeling energy—you are not prepared to manipulate energy in any way until you receive personal training.

Simply learning to feel energy will reward your efforts, for it will start a conscious flow between you and the things around you. Without manipulating energy you will still be helping your own energy flow in ways you may not have noticed before.

Aromatherapy

It is important to respect essential oils if you choose to use them. Oils are eight times more potent than similar conventional medicines and can over-whelm the body if improperly used. Rose oil is specifically used on Fourth Chakra issues, but also for Fourth Chakra illnesses. Typically the use of Rose oil is combined with a Reflexology application: mix 1 tsp vegetable oil (can substitute grapeseed oil or almond oil) and one drop of Rose oil into palm of hand; rub hands together lightly and then massage the oil mixture onto the bottoms of the client's feet, with special attention given to the left foot (under the ball of the big toe just above the instep), do not rub for more than ten seconds.

Rose oil opens you to processing for-giveness and grief. Many people have been known to cry when exposed to rose oil (and not just be-cause they remember a date who brought roses and then broke their heart). The scent of roses is also said to be sensed when one is visited by The Holy Mother Mary, and in the blood of people with the marks of the Stigmata. It is probably no coincidence that rose oil is linked to the heart chakra, or that the heart chakra is home for the soul.

\\\\

Reflexology

This technique may also be called acupressure, but it is different because it is focused on mirroring the body's organ systems in the feet and hands (but many reflexologists also "massage" the shoulders, neck and head). The "heart" is located on your left foot (but you can also "treat" your right foot) below the ball of the big toe and slightly toward the center of the foot above the arch.

The heart point on the hands is mainly on the left hand (but you can mirror it on the right hand if so desired). It is between the "mounds" (or knuckles below the fingers and above the thumb), in the center of the palm of the hand but closer to the left edge (thumb side) than the exact center of the palm.

Putting pressure on any organ point that is experiencing a "problem" may result in tenderness, sometimes to the point of pain. It is important to still put pressure on the point, but you may want to start with a lighter pressure than you use on other points. The goal is to release toxins, not to cause pain.

When you apply pressure to any point in reflexology you don't want to do so for more than 9 seconds (but I have seen some sources that say 15 seconds). You can simply put constant pressure on the point you choose, or make tiny circular motions with your finger on the point. If you choose to do both feet (and both hands) you don't want your overall treatment to take more than 20 minutes; more will overload the body with the toxins you are releasing and make the recipient nauseous (diarrhea and headaches are also common). Regardless of how long your session is, drinking water after is always recommended. It helps to flush the released toxins from the body (so does sweating, urination, etc.).

Using rose oil during a reflexology treatment will provide twice the desired effect, but means that twice the toxic release may be required, so ensure fluid intake.

Prayer

There is not much difference between being in a constant state of prayer (or communication with the Universe) and being an intuitive. It is like an internal dialog you have but it is not one-sided. You may not hear voices, but if you pay close attention you will get answers to the questions you ask or comments you make.

It is important to pray for the people

you love and for the ones you will never know or meet. There is an energy to prayer though so it is best to ensure you pray with a sense of gratitude rather than need. Of course since God knows your heart and is the closest being you will ever talk with, you can be honest with Him. He is there for your venting and for your praise.

There was a time in my life that I stopped praying. It was a lonely time for me but I was stuck with a concern and could not figure out a way around it. I became afraid of the way I was praying, not all of the time but for special requests. I would pass a hitchhiker and pray, "God please bless his journey." It sounds innocent enough, but when I thought about it, it sounded accusatory—like I was telling God He was slipping on the job. It also had a flair of arrogance, as if He needed my permission to reach out to that person. It may sound foolish to you, but to me it was a problem that got bigger with time.

The more I tried to change what I prayed, the worse it got. When I hear sirens I try to consistently pray for the people involved—victims, perpetrators, families, onlookers and response personnel. They all flash through my mind as I pray, "Please God, bless their journeys according to their greater good." I thought mentioning their greater good and asking please would alleviate some of the arrogance, but I still could not get past the accusation. I wanted to find a way to add my blessings (energy) to the situation without being offensive. Permanently quitting prayer was not an option, but praying was causing me great concern.

Of course because I had such a habit of constant communication with God, He was whom I went to for answers. I did not feel any cause for concern coming from Him, but my inner being was still upset. That started a long succession of experiments, but finally I reached a prayer that provided me with peace while making my wishes known. Now when I hear a siren I simply pray, "Lord, please add my energy to their journey." We have an understanding that the "their" is all-inclusive of everyone involved or witnessing, and that the energy being added is positive and supportive (for the greater good of all concerned).

Note that adding your energy forms a connection from you to the situation at hand; it is important to cut that connection, and to be aware of your own energy levels. If you are depleted or struggling with a health issue perhaps it's wiser to pray: "Lord, please add my blessings to their journey." Even though I may have indicated that blessings and energy are the same (blessings are energy), giving direct energy connects you; giving a blessing (which is energy), or money (which is energy), allows you to disconnect without effort.

There is a difference between constant inner dialog and prayer. The inner dialog is time spent with an unconditional friend (which is God, your Guides and other holy entities you wish to include) which is not filtered or filled with agenda; prayer is time spent with God. It is more structured and has a goal of voicing your concerns and issuing your desires and blessings.

The difference between prayer and meditation is that the first is talking and the latter is listening—I like to listen during prayer too, but then it turns into more of a dialog. Meditation is calming your mind; losing yourself in quiet and solitude; opening yourself to whatever comes.

There are also guided meditations

designed to take your mind on a "visual" trip; this kind of meditation can provide you with answers and is usually meant to bring some kind of understanding (even if that is to learn how to relax or take a short mental break).

There is a reverence during prayer because we are talking with our Creator, but the God I love and worship wants us to also have a personal relationship with Him. Regardless of how you view communication with God, it is energetically important to participate in it especially if you believe that intuition has a spiritual source.

Why would I tell you any of this? There is a risk when you start talking about intimate spiritual details with others. I simply want you to know that it is okay to have doubts and dilemmas and second guessing because at the root of it all is the fact that you are curious, adventurous, and on a mission to uncover secrets that will bring you even closer to your Creator. You truly do not have to be worried about right and wrong, moral and sinful, legitimate and falsified. Pray that you will find the path and it will be presented to you.

It muddies the waters to say that in praying for peace you will be delivered chaos, for what other way can you know peace except through experiencing chaos? Suffice it to say that you will learn how to pray, sometimes through trial and error. If you have concerns discuss them with your pastor. But prayer is good because it helps you to unload the burdens on your soul and to vent some of your internal pressure.

Gratitude

We cannot leave the topic of prayer without mentioning gratitude. It is important to pray with gratitude in your heart. If your world is falling down around you, try to find something positive for which you can thank God. He knows your needs and challenges, and yes, He does enjoy you expressing your needs, but if that is all He hears…well, have you ever tried to have a discussion with a whiny child? No matter what you say or how you try to divert the child's attention the situation just seems to get worse. God loves us, but do you wonder sometimes what your prayers sound like to Him?

If I am allowed to awaken to a quiet house instead of a phone call, the first words I say (or think) are: "Thank you. Thank you God for this beautiful day." This is before I check the weather or the schedule or look for any gifts the animals have left on the carpet, because I know that whatever the day holds, I go with God, and that makes it a good day. Sure, I may fortify myself with some jewelry or a specially colored outfit, but that is just a tool belt to prepare me for the job ahead.

Think about it, if all your child did was whine and demand—the same old record every time you tried to have a discussion—wouldn't you lose interest or attempt to avoid talking? No, I'm not inferring that God mirrors this human reaction in any way, but you would be dealing with one child (or perhaps more), what if you had billions whining, demanding and otherwise throwing tantrums? That one small voice offering you praise, or a laugh and a simple "thank you," might be just the respite needed to give you hope (that the others might also learn to be grateful).

Compliments

You are going to wonder if I follow my own advice (e.g. from Third Chakra discussion earlier), but I am going to encourage you to give others compliments. Why would

I do that after insisting that you elevate your energy above the entrapping energy of compliments? We do not know what kind of day the people we encounter have had. We do not know if there is anyone who cares enough to give them a kind word or a smile. Whether that person is a child, an adult, a boss, a customer, an official, and yes, even a telemarketer, a kind word of praise goes a long way.

You do have to give the compliment without hidden agenda, other than that there are no rules. Sure, some of the compliments you give may not be the most sincere, some may sound like you are patronizing the recipient, but do not concern yourself with details. Simply teach yourself the routine of finding something good in the people you come in contact with, and let them know you noticed. After a while it will become a part of your nature to make a kind remark and it will be sincere. Their hearts will benefit and so will yours.

Laughter

Laugh hard and laugh often. Your

soul needs to feel joy. Will it get you into trouble sometimes? Most certainly. I have been chastised by more than one child for laughing when they "…could have been hurt really bad." I have a weakness for slapstick comedy, and well, some five-year-olds cannot catch a ball without fumbling it up into their faces, or through their legs. It is just too cute to watch without laughing.

When I drop something loudly in a quiet room, I have to laugh. Sure, stubbing my toe may not be met with an immediate laugh, but after the initial pain wave passes I have to laugh at how clumsy I am.

Have there been embarrassing moments caused by my laughing? If you ever talked with my sister you would know there certainly have been, but I would not trade one of those moments of perfect enjoyment for anything. And, when there is not anything to laugh about, because trauma does come to us all, we talk about those times we laughed with loved ones who have ascended, and we smile (or laugh all over again).

If you do not have a person to share laughter with, movies or comedy shows can be a suitable substitute. It does not matter

what causes you to laugh (as long as you are
not a psychopath laughing only at others'
pain), it is just important that you do laugh.

The laughs that are the best are the
deep, guttural ones that shake your whole
body and bring tears to your eyes—these
laughs serve to cleanse your body and balance your chakras. However, any laughter is
better than none at all.

Charity

It is said, "You can't take it with you." No
one can, but we store up things while we are here as
if it was possible to leave the planet with them. The
fact of the matter is that we are merely stewards for
the matter we collect and the energy we attract.
Wealth is an energy, and one way we can ensure we
attract wealth is to share the wealth we attract to us.

The fear of losing something is what chokes
the energy out of it and kills its ability to thrive.
Have you ever noticed that the people who have the
least are the most apt to share what they have? People with more are more focused with how to protect
assets. They have more to lose so they fear others'
agendas. That kind of fear attracts loss.

One way to ensure you keep attracting

abundance is to willingly share. Energy is attracted by flow, and God is the ultimate recycler. When He knows He can trust you with multiplying His gifts He will continue to bless you. A giving heart is a guarantee of riches beyond imagination. You may have times when you do not know what the next day will bring, but as long as you continue to give (of whatever you have to offer) you will continue to be blessed by receiving. God does not want anyone to do without. He feels our pain and knows our needs and delights in our generosities.

Forgiveness

One of the primary functions of heart energy is to help us with forgiveness. Many people have a hard time believing they have not dealt with past issues and that old, pent up energy is corroding their systems. Venting is a way to release your feelings, but if you are still venting over that opportunity you missed twenty years ago, you have a problem with forgiveness. Whether it is another person, an organization, or yourself that you need to forgive does not matter. Your inability to forgive (or let go) results in bitterness and stress on your heart chakra and the systems it supports.

One way to investigate whether or not your history has the better of you is to ask those close to you how often you bring up past events, and in what light you paint those events. Do you tend to rant or rave about things beyond your control and out of your (present) time zone? Would you need a time machine to right the wrongs that occupy most of your thought and conversation?

Admittedly, there are traumatic events some of us are asked to endure and it may not seem fair at times. But, just because it seems like others have it easy does not mean it is so. Just as others cannot truly know the pain you feel inside, it is impossible for you to truly know another's pain. You can ask yourself a question though: "Is it worth it?" What do you gain by keeping your pain? What do you gain by carrying hate and bitterness in your heart besides poor health and the possibility of a much shorter life? Every one of us has to learn how to forgive; it is a challenge of being human.

We ask God to forgive us, and in turn we are expected to mirror His grace. The forgiveness we give to our fellow humans is not of the caliber we receive from God though. God has the power to absolve our transgressions. We do not have such power. The people we forgive will still have to do penance with everyone concerned before they can be at peace.

When someone has wronged you and you

feel powerless to cope with the injury, you can turn the entire event over to God. You do not have to confront the person who hurt you; God helps by taking that burden from you. God promises you that He will resolve things with the ones who have wronged you. What better warrior could you have in your corner? You do not have to be concerned with the details, you have only to live your life to the fullest and be as far removed from the trauma as possible. If it helps you might carry the mantra, "What goes around comes around," to empower your efforts to forgive.

Perhaps it will help if you remember that forgiving someone doesn't condone what they did. Forgiveness is the act of taking that pain from you and turning it over to God to process. God has had centuries more experience dealing with the deeds of man; He knows best how to deal with transgressions, and how to reach the heart of the specific person (or issue) you have brought to Him. "Vengeance is Mine, sayeth the Lord." Romans 12:19.

Keeping Promises

A promise is a contract. Intentionally breaking a promise is the equivalent of lying and costs you energy. The more you fail to keep promises the greater your energetic debt. The greater that debt becomes the more it evolves into more serious repercussions. People start to distrust you; your word no longer means anything. You become a disappointment.

We are imperfect creatures living in an imperfect world, so there are bound to be times that you simply cannot meet all of your obligations. That is okay and is certainly forgivable. But, if you know ahead of time that you will not be able to honor a request, then you should not make a promise to do so. At most you might promise to *try*, but people listen selectively and probably will not hear any reservations on your part. If there is a chance you will not be able to do what another is requesting, then own up to that even if it costs you an awkward moment. It is better for someone to be angry with you because you say, "No," than it is for someone to be counting on you to deliver something you have no intentions of delivering.

You may get by with lax promise making for a while. A few profuse apologies may smooth the ruffled feathers at first, but if you consistently let people down they will see you for the selfish person you are being. Emotional walls will be built and if situations are serious enough the battle begins. You may not even see it coming because it has a subtle start. At first there may be giggles and IOUs, then maybe a few short words, the next failure may bring tears or yelling, and it will not be long after that that character bashing will start.

Just as feuds escalate, so do bad feelings—you start out as friends and become bitter enemies. You have succeeded in making someone hate you, which does not serve either of you. You will feel the energetic harpoons that are being tossed at you, and it will cost you just as much energy to return fire. This may be amusing for a while, but over time it will physically cost you, and most of it will make a direct hit on your heart chakra.

Another variety of this push and pull between people is when one does all of the giving and the other does all of the taking. Eventually, the giver is drained dry and has nothing left to offer the taker. If you are afraid you may be a taker, take a hard look at your ability to keep promises (or to put others first).

If you want to keep your promises, pay attention to what you say to others; do not bite off more than you can chew. Do not sacrifice your physical safety by trying to be the good guy all of the time or by telling people what you think they want to hear. Perhaps a part of your contract is to learn how to be honest with others, and that involves being able to step in and help when you can, and backing down when you know you cannot.

Relaxation

Sure, in this instant gratification, get it done now world, how does anyone make time to relax? Then when you do there are a dozen things to do in order to get ready to relax (e.g. extra shopping, lugging stuff around, inviting people, fixing food). All of the work required seems to make the effort of relaxing exhausting. Of course there is always television or home movies, but they may not help the mind shut down. There is also the bombardment of electrical waves produced by computers and televisions (and the dozens of electrical items we have running at any given time) that can cause us to become more agitated than relaxed.

Hobbies are wonderful, but some are expensive which may cause hesitation to participate or stress when you do. Some people look forward to a long bubble bath at the end of a long week. Some people prefer to relax with family and friends, some crave an evening alone.

It does not matter what you have to go through to get relaxation, it only matters that you have some time set aside to breathe, quiet your mind, and give your soul a chance to marvel at the world around you. There are no set rules, it may only take you a few seconds, or it might take you a week. You may be able to sneak those moments when you play a game with a child, or you may feel like you need to fly away to an island resort. The point is to reconnect with that special essence inside of you that makes you who you are. It is a quiet, soft, timeless moment meant to realign your being in peace and serenity. It allows that small part of God whom lives in each of us an opportunity to say, "Ahhh."

Quiet Time

Similar to relaxation, but oh so different is the need for quiet time. In relaxation you are merely escaping "work;" in quiet time you are escaping the world around you. Relaxation can be done in a crowd, but quiet time involves the aspect of solitude (even though it can be accomplished within a crowd).

We need time to disconnect from all of the drains on our energy and to simply "be." Of course if you are the parent of a young child you are probably laughing through your tears right now. How could I suggest such a thing? We actually store up extra energy to get through such times, so rest assured that you will get through the sparse times. Unfortunately, what happens to us is that as the demand on our full attention lessons, we tend to fill the void with even more demand.

It helps if we come to realize how important investing our precious minutes into quiet time can truly be to our psyche, spirit and body. Have you ever had a problem, or something you have not quite figured out or decided, and then, in the shower you have the most brilliant revelation? Perhaps it was the rhythm of the water or the relaxing steam but you were lured into a quiet space with just you and your thoughts (and you were probably not thinking about much). What brought you into the quiet zone is not important; being there is what is important.

Granted, we all have those three-minute showers that are more tedium than relaxation because we are already running behind in our schedule, so we cannot depend on hygiene moments to count as our personal time. Quiet time is set aside for us to not have to be anything to anybody else. It is time that each one of us can claim as our own.

If you are a gardener you know how important the alone time is that you have to commune with nature (so you may not have to set aside more time to be quiet). But if you use that time to fret over things rather than letting your mind rest then you may as well be in a corporate board meeting.

Quiet time does not require a structure. It is just as beneficial if you steal a bit of time here or there as it is if you write it into your schedule. As long as you find some time to simply let your mind be as blank as it chooses to be.

Life Meets Chakra

Since stress is one of the causes of heart dis-ease I would be remiss if I did not at least mention some of the stressors that we run into as we progress through the years. I will not discuss them, but I will make a short list of the chakras that carry the primary burden for the energetic interchanges that accompany the physical and emotional occurrences more commonly experienced. Yes, this is another list, and as you may have guessed it carries the caveat that it is not all-inclusive; feel free to add your own events and if needed, you can refer back to the chakra section to determine which chakras may be involved.

You will note that more than one chakra is listed for the events. The first one listed is the primary target for a loss of energy. Remember that the chakras are interrelated, with shared emotions running through them, so it stands to reason that you may process energetic stress in more than one location. What do I mean? When an event happens it will be sent to the chakra handling that energy for processing. If the stress of that emotion is too big for one chakra to handle without becoming "bankrupt" then other chakras will be tapped for energetic resupply and/or the emotion itself will travel to a different chakra for processing. Sometimes that sharing between the chakras will facilitate energy conservation, and sometimes it will be because that emotion (at least for the current event) is supposed to be processed by a different chakra.

For example, Vickie's dog died. Of course she loved the dog, but she had more of a business relationship with the dog than an emotional one. The dog was a member of the family, but a well-trained member who lived out in the garage. Vickie and the dog visited hospitals throughout the state and Vickie used the dog to help train other animals for "buddy" certifications. When the dog died she found that while she did have a short period of grief, her bigger need was to replace the dog so she could continue her work. Vickie's greatest apprehension after the death of her dog was whether she could replace it with one as gentle and friendly. So, in Vickie's situation her grief over the loss of her dog is really more of grief over the loss of part of her identity. In her situation she may experience more demand on her 3rd Chakra (Ego) than on her 4th Chakra (Heart).

Where you experience a huge loss of energy may not be where someone else does. Knowing your own physical and emotional feelings is important to ensure you use the information you are learning to your best advantage. What do I mean? Just because the book says competitiveness and personal finances are 2nd Chakra issues does not mean that you will automatically process the loss of a promotion primarily in the 2nd Chakra. If you had set your dreams on that job since you were a small child you may have true passion for earning the opportunity to be a success in that job. Your emotional intensity may be so completely attached to the 4th Chakra that you grieve over the loss of the promotion as if it were a deceased loved one.

Think of your chakra system as a chain of banks belonging to the same company. Each bank (chakra) is provided with the same amount of funds (energy) to have on hand to cover the overhead and handle emergencies. The banks (chakras) in the chain quite frequently share funds (energy) among each other to keep the balance between them as equal as possible. Then one of the banks starts to receive more withdrawals than it has had in the past—it is not prepared for the extra demand, so it calls the other banks for funds.

The banks (chakras) who respond are the ones with more expertise to handle the needs of the customers (emotions needing processing), so instead of just shifting funds the banks decide to shift the clientele. This provides balance for a while but if the demands keep coming the hardest hit of the banks in the chain experience deficits that the other banks cannot handle. The chain has to get public support (from organs/systems); it goes to the area of most demand and requests donations from the residents.

Since the residents (organs) still get support from that local bank, they provide the assets they can. This puts a plug in the immediate drain of energy, and for a while the chain of banks recovers. But, when the books are balanced (chakras are balanced) the next month the chain discovers that there is still unprecedented demand on the one bank and the rest of the chain has still not recovered enough to provide support.

The only choice left is for the area residents to take over the bank and provide it with all of the funds needed to keep it open, even though the residents will have to sacrifice their own well-being. If the demand continues after this point some of the area residents may have to be cut off from bank support—this means that the deprived area will be weak and compromised and subject to take over from enemy agents (organs/systems depleted of necessary energy will succumb to dis-ease).

Simple, yes, but representative of how our internal energy system works. We are given several opportunities to replenish our energy stores. We are also provided with ample deliveries to keep all of the customers happy—until demand overwhelms the system. The quicker we pay our emotional bills the faster we balance our books.

You know yourself. Trust your instincts if you feel emotional energies belong somewhere else in your chakral system.

Then, translate that information into the physical system that will be paying for your emotional deficits. As long as you realize that your emotional health has an impact on your physical health, and visa versa, you are ahead of the game. You can augment your diet to support physical systems, etc., and you can process emotions; both of which provide energy to your chakras and balance to your being.

To start you on your journey of discovery, here is a list of chakras I would suspect the following events to process through. Remember, in some cases the primary chakra (first one listed) may be as far as you need to go. In other cases you may skip the first chakra I list and go to another one on the list (or to another one altogether), or you may have to go through all of them to fully process the issue.

Regardless of which chakra you are working with, bear in mind that all decisions (for feeling, action, investment of energy, etc.) are approved by the Heart Chakra first, so even if another chakra has primary lead on a certain issue, the Heart Chakra will be touched. I may not list the 4th Chakra in every case, but you might have more heart energy invested than the average person, or your situation may engage the heart more than another's situation.

This list can apply to any health situation you are experiencing. I developed it to be generic and the chakras matched to it to be from a broad point of view. What do I mean? Suppose you were processing the "loss of a job" entry; you could be looking at it as a boss experiencing the guilt of having to lay off 100 people or as a person losing a sole source of income. The chakras I have listed are meant to handle a broad spectrum of situations within each topic.

Death of a loved one: 4, 2, 1

Marriage: 4, 2, 6, 1, 3, 5, 7

Divorce: 2, 4, 1, 3

Loss of a job: 2, 1, 3

New job; change in employment: 3, 6, 5, 1, 2

Elderly parent; special needs family member: 1, 4, 2, 5

Health crisis: 6, 1, 4, 2

Loved one in hospital: 1, 4, 2

Financial concerns: 2, 1, 6

Adult education: 3, 6, 2

Children leaving home; starting school: 2, 4, 1, 6

Spiritual identity crisis: 4, 5, 7, 6

Creative blocks: 2, 6, 4, 5

Career frustration: 3, 6, 2

Family feuds: 1, 5, 4

Teenage anxieties: 3, 6, 5, 2, 1

Teenage pregnancy/relationships: 2, 3, 1, 6, 4

Fertility concerns: 2, 4, 1, 6, 7

Pregnancy options/concerns: 6, 4, 2, 1, 5

Birth defects: 4, 1, 6, 5, 7, 3

Abortion: 2, 4, 1, 6

Crime: 1, 2, 3, 5, 6, 4

Victimization: 2, 3, 1, 4

Loss of home: 3, 1, 2

Catastrophic accident/natural disaster: 1, 4, 2, 6

Romantic crush: 2, 4, 3

Failed romance: 4, 2, 5, 7, 1

Stolen project: 3, 5, 1, 2

Distressed workplace: 2, 3, 6, 5, 1

Homelessness: 1, 3, 5

Starvation: 1, 2, 7, 6, 4, 5

Alcoholism: 2, 1, 3, 5

Drug addiction/addiction: 2, 1, 3, 5

Depression: 4, 3, 5, 2, 1, 6

Procreation angst: 2, 3, 4, 1

Business contracts: 6, 3, 5

Technology frustration: 6, 5, 3, 1

Dieting: 2, 5, 3, 1, 4

Moving: 2, 1, 4, 6, 5

Buying a house: 6, 4, 3, 1

Witness protection: 4, 1, 5, 2

Abandonment: 4, 1, 3, 2, 5, 6

Paying bills: 2, 1, 3, 5, 6

Major investments: 6, 5, 2, 1, 4

Long-term commitments: 4, 2, 6, 5, 3

Bullies: 4, 5, 1, 3

Homework:

1. Make a list of the energy work topics you would like to explore, if needed visit your library or bookstore and see which books you are energetically attracted to
2. If I have left out a topic (energy, chakra, physical ailment) you want to know more about, then conduct your research and take notes
3. If you have additions to the lists above or other places in the book, then ensure you document them and explore them because they were given to you for a reason
4. Start working on your own dialog with the Universe, the more you work with energy the more you will have to say
5. As ludicrous, simple, or silly as some of the energy work suggestions are, pick one and try it out for a week and see if you can feel a difference; then, if you want to dig deeper try some books on meditation, dream incubation/analysis, medical intuition, past-life, near-death experience, self-healing, energy medicine, or anything that attracts you in the

alternative healthcare section of your bookstore or library

6. Experiment with the Life Meets Chakra list; pick a topic that you have experienced in the past and go through the chakras listed (refer to the emotions and physical systems each pertains to); take notes on how you emotionally processed that situation and compare it to how you feel the chakras line up; explore any health issues that may have resulted from the topic you chose (if there were any, you probably have more than one encounter with that topic to explore)

7. Explore your current situation for a topic that you may be emotionally involved with now and see how it is affecting your system; use your chakra information to help you through, knowing that this is one more tool for you to use to help you maintain harmony

In closing, thank you for allowing me a chance to offer you a starting place for your exploration into energy medicine. There are many authors and teachers available to help you on your path, if you seek you shall find.

Just remember that conventional medicine shouldn't be ignored. If you are under a doctor's care please do your best to follow guidance. If you have suggestions to add to your healthcare regimen based on your research and/or intuition, discuss them with your provider.

You'd be amazed how receptive conventional medicine has become toward alternative concepts

HEART STRINGS

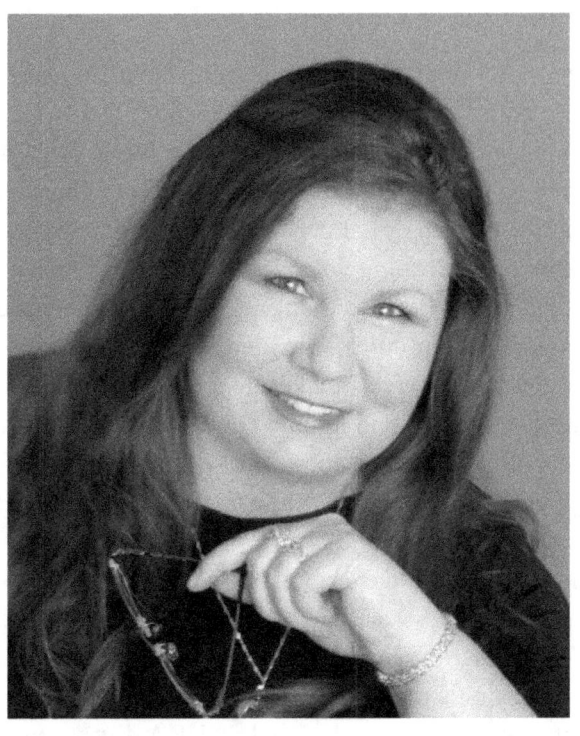

Linda Marie received her Ph.D. in Energy Medicine from Universal University of Holistic Spirituality in July, 2005, and earned her doctorate in theology with honors from Holos University Graduate Seminary in Springfield, MO, in September 2004. Her dissertation study was conducted on The Effects of Archetype Education and Analysis on Depression. Prior to that she studied archetypes and medical intuition for almost five years with Drs. Caroline Myss and C. Norman Shealy. She is a certified aromatherapist, a Reiki master, and has completed multiple levels of Pranic Healing while dabbling in self-study in many other energy medicine modalities. Before gravitating toward energy healing interests, Linda was a business executive in the *serious* world of government with responsibility for hundreds of subordinates and multi-million dollar accounts. She has twenty years of experience working with many different world cultures and ethnic groups, along with people from varied economic backgrounds—the kind of exposure to life situations that she feels makes her more energetically open in her work as an intuitive and spiritual consultant. Clients of Linda's rave about her open and non-judgmental approach to helping them get in touch with their emotional pain and behavior blocks. In addition to doing archetype and energy work with people, Linda continues to study relationships. In the spare time she had during her previous career, Linda was also a wife, divorcee, single mother, grandmother of a terminally ill infant, cancer patient, advanced SCUBA diver, equestrian, Girl Scout troop assistant leader, church choir leader, Bible school teacher, fashion designer, interior decorator, author of an unpublished romance-adventure novel, student earning a master's degree in business, community theater actor, writer/producer/director/actor in several organizational productions, and the proud owner of a loud cackle of a laugh that has gotten her in trouble on more than one occasion. She currently lives in Kansas, but considers herself a world citizen.